THE SCIENCE OF AMERICAN FOOTBALL

T0386162

The game of American football may be the greatest team sport that exists. It epitomizes the need of a "team" first approach to achieve the desired success. Success is often measured as the hoisting of a championship trophy, which involved a journey that required discipline, perseverance, sacrifice, and hard work. These traits are the backbone of success in football, but more importantly they are the backbone or blueprint for success in life.

The Science of American Football provides an in-depth discussion on the physiology of the game of American football, including the physiological strain associated with playing in various environmental extremes. Acclimatization, preparation, and medical issues associated with each of these environmental extremes are discussed as well as the medical issues occurring during the athlete's playing career (common sites of injury) and potential risks arising post-career (e.g. neurological dysfunction, arthritic joints, obesity).

The book goes on to consider aspects of player selection and preparation, including discussion of evidence-based physical conditioning programs, appropriate nutrition, and specific dietary supplementation for the American football player.

The Science of American Football is the first book to focus on the physiology, science, and medical issues associated with the game of American football and will be key reading for students of coaching and exercise science as well as those with a keen interest in understanding the science of American football, such as coaches and players.

Jay R. Hoffman is a professor in the Physical Therapy Department at Ariel University in Israel. He is also Head Coach of Israel's National American Football Team. He is a fellow of the American College of Sports Medicine and has previously served as President of the Board of the National Strength and Conditioning Association (NSCA) and on the Board of the US Bobsled and Skeleton Federation. Prior to his academic career, he signed free agent contracts with the New York Jets and Philadelphia Eagles of the NFL and the Tampa Bay Bandits of the USFL.

THE SCIENCE OF AMERICAN FOOTBALL

Jay R. Hoffman

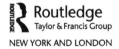

Routledge
Taylor & Francis Group

NEW YORK AND LONDON

First published 2021
by Routledge
52 Vanderbilt Avenue, New York, NY 10017

and by Routledge
2 Park Square, Milton Park, Abingdon, Oxon, OX14 4RN

Routledge is an imprint of the Taylor & Francis Group, an informa business

© 2021 Taylor & Francis

Library of Congress Cataloging-in-Publication Data
Names: Hoffman, Jay, 1961– author.
Title: The science of American football / Jay R. Hoffman.
Description: New York, NY : Routledge, 2020. | Includes bibliographical
    references and index.
Identifiers: LCCN 2020037450 (print) | LCCN 2020037451 (ebook) |
    ISBN 9780367462833 (hardback) | ISBN 9780367462710 (paperback) |
    ISBN 9781003027881 (ebook)
Subjects: LCSH: Football—Physiological aspects. | Football injuries. | Football
    players—Nutrition. | Football—Coaching.
Classification: LCC RC1220.F6 H638 2020 (print) | LCC RC1220.F6 (ebook) |
    DDC 617.1/027332—dc23
LC record available at https://lccn.loc.gov/2020037450
LC ebook record available at https://lccn.loc.gov/2020037451

ISBN: 978-0-367-46283-3 (hbk)
ISBN: 978-0-367-46271-0 (pbk)
ISBN: 978-1-003-02788-1 (ebk)

Typeset in Bembo
by Apex CoVantage, LLC

CONTENTS

FIGURES

TABLES

PREFACE

The game of American football may be the greatest team sport that exists. It epitomizes the need of a "team" first approach to achieve the desired success. Success is often measured as the hoisting of a championship trophy, be it a conference championship, league championship, bowl game, or Super Bowl. The memories of the championship or of a successful season may be represented by a ring, trophy, or other memorabilia piece of jewelry. However, the scores and memories of the season often fade, but it is the life's lessons learned that will always be remembered. Football is a unique game in which there is only a very small window of opportunity that permits an athlete to play the game. It is a sport, unlike other team sports such as basketball, baseball, soccer, or even ice hockey, that does not permit a recreational version to be played years after the competitive version has been retired. The lessons of the game are not always clear during the athlete's career, but as the former player finds success in other endeavors in their lives, they recognize that the traits that resulted in their success were first learned while playing the game of football. Teamwork, discipline, perseverance, sacrifice, and hard work are the hallmark traits and backbone of success in football. But more importantly these traits are also the backbone or blueprint for success in life.

This blueprint for success is not dependent upon the innate ability of an athlete to be a great football player. Even the least talented football player in a team will still benefit from the "lessons of the game" and use these lessons for success in many other of life's endeavors. The lessons learned are the ticket earned to find success. It is similar to the Ph.D. degree – a degree of persistence and a degree that is actually a key that unlocks a door to possibility and potential but does not guarantee anything except the chance to still compete. It is what one does with their Ph.D. degree that determines whether they are a good scientist or not, but by itself it is an indicator of persistence only. Likewise, the "lessons of the game" is the starting point for success in football. This book begins with the point that the athlete is disciplined, ready to sacrifice personal glory for team success, and willing to work hard. It focuses on the science behind the sport. It details physiological limitations, adaptations, medical issues during and following the athlete's career, and how coaching can both positively and negatively impact player success.

ACKNOWLEDGEMENTS

Success is not achieved independently, but is a collaborative effort of strong support, tremendous guidance and people that are willing to share their expertise as you partake in the journey of life. None of what I have been able to accomplish would be possible without my wife Yaffa, and the support of my children Raquel, Mattan and Ariel. They are my strength. My love of the game of football was set at an early age by my father, Lewis, who taught me many things in life but no one else could have taught me the value of a good "forearm shiver".

I also would like to acknowledge the coaches and players who I had the honor of working for, with and coached, who all contributed in important ways to my development as a coach and sport scientist. Special acknowledgement to Coach Eric Hamilton at The College of New Jersey who not only was a tremendous coach, but understood the importance that science can have on enhancing the players' ability to reach their football playing potential. The eight years that I was on his staff was unbelievably rewarding. Finally, the scores may have been forgotten, but the memory of the players that I have coached does not fade. The greatest reward that comes from coaching is the impact that you can make on a young man's life, and the impact that this has on your own. Always take a step back and enjoy that moment, it is the small treasures that life has to offer that makes the difference!

Yours in football,

1

PHYSIOLOGY OF AMERICAN FOOTBALL

Introduction

Despite football being one of the most popular sports in North America, whose global out-reach is growing stronger every year, the scientific understanding of the game is less than any of the other major sports such as soccer, basketball, or even baseball. This is likely related to the relatively low number of games played during the season and the inability to simulate a game or have a practice game for the benefit of scientific discovery. In addition, the imaginary wall between academics and athletics across college campuses around the nation has unfortunately limited the degree of collaboration. As such, the ability to study football players during an actual competitive event has been very limited.

The vast majority of research in American football has focused on the physical requirements of the game. Research of the past 30 years has clearly demonstrated the importance of strength, power, and speed at all competitive levels (Berg et al., 1990; Black and Roundy, 1994; Fry and Kraemer, 1991; Garstecki et al., 2004; Kraemer and Gotshalk, 2000). Investigations have shown that strength, power, and speed can differentiate starters from nonstarters and may also differ-entiate athletes between different levels of competition (Berg et al., 1990; Fry and Kraemer, 1991; Kraemer and Gotshalk, 2000). The evidence from these investigations has assisted football coaches and scouts regarding the type of athlete to recruit and has also generated a degree of scientific curiosity for sport scientists to examine various training paradigms and their potential effect on improving athletic performance in football players (Hoffman et al., 2004a, 2005a, 2009a). Performance improvements in college football players appear to occur in the early part of the athlete's playing career (Hoffman et al., 2011; Miller et al., 2002), with a much lower rate of improvement observed in subsequent years. This will be covered in greater detail in Chapter 3.

Physiological Demands of American Football

The number of physiological studies conducted on the sport of American football is very limited in comparison to the large body of work on strength, power, or speed development. The separa-tion often seen between sport science and university athletic programs, especially at the National Collegiate Athletic Association (NCAA) Division I level within the United States, is likely in part responsible for this paucity of data (Hoffman, 2015). But there are many other reasons as well, including the lack of appreciation for the potential contributions that sport science can make, the limited access to conduct invasive procedures (e.g., blood draws or muscle biopsies), and an inability of the research team to conduct a field study. There have only been a limited number of studies that have examined the physiological stress of a game or a competitive season. Much of our understanding regarding the physiological requirements of the game is based primarily on empirical evidence. Recently, technological advancements have provided a noninvasive approach (i.e., global positioning systems [GPS]) to examining specific movement patterns of football players during competition, which has helped further our understanding and has increased our ability to determine physiological and metabolic demands placed on these athletes.

The Game of Football

There are 22 athletes on the field at all times. Eleven of those athletes play offense, while the other 11 athletes play defense. The overall goal of the offense is to score: Whether it is touchdown in which an offensive player carries the ball across the goal line, which is worth six points, or they kick a field goal, which is worth three points. After a touchdown, the offense can kick an extra point worth one point, or attempt to score (run or pass) the ball from the 3-yard line into the end zone for two points. The offensive team comprises five linemen (two tackles, two guards, and a center). The responsibility of the center is to snap the ball to the quarterback. The guards line up on either side of the center, while the tackles are positioned on the outside shoulder of the guards. All five of these linemen are generally in a three-point stance. There are certain instances when the guards and tackles may be in a two-point stance with their hands on their thighs. These athletes are generally the bigger players on the field whose primary responsibility is to protect the quarterback when he passes the ball, or block for the running backs as they run the ball. The other players on the offensive side of the ball are considered to be "skill position players" and include a quarterback, whose responsibilities include calling the plays, passing the ball, or running with the ball. The quarterback is expected to be the leader of the offense. He is given the play by the coach and has the responsibility to run that play or decide based upon the defensive alignment that a different play may be more appropriate. This decision-making requirement adds a significant cognitive load to the quarterback. The other skill position players include one or two running backs and three or four wide receivers. Running backs have several responsibilities that include taking a hand-off from the quarterback and running the ball. They may also be required to catch the ball when it is thrown, and they may also have blocking responsibilities. The wide receivers generally are required to catch the ball when it is thrown by the quarterback and block during running plays. They are generally the faster athletes on the offensive team. One of the receivers may be a tight end. He lines up next to one of the tackles on the outside shoulder (hence the term "tight") and is generally a bigger athlete who has greater blocking responsibility than the other receivers. The other receivers generally line up away from the linemen (hence the term "wide"). The skill position players generally begin the play in a two-point stance; however, the tight end often lines up in a three-point stance.

On the defensive side of the ball, the positional composition of the team can vary depending upon the schemes of the coach, or in response to the substitution pattern of the offense. In general, the defense consists of a combination of three to four defensive linemen, three to four linebackers, and four to five defensive backs. The goal for each defensive player is to react to what the offense is attempting to do and prevent the offense from scoring. The defense also has the ability to score a touchdown from either intercepting a pass and running it into the end zone or recovering a fumble (e.g., a ball that is knocked away from one of the offensive skill position players) and running the fumble into the end zone. Defensive linemen are generally in a three-point stance and are positioned either "head-up" or "shaded" to either the inside or the outside shoulder of an offensive lineman. They position themselves as close to the line of scrimmage (e.g., where the ball is placed) as possible. The linebackers are generally positioned 5 yards off the ball and are in a two-point stance. The defensive backs are often divided into cornerbacks and safeties. The cornerbacks are responsible for covering the fastest players on the field – the wide receivers, while the safeties will also cover wide receivers, but they may also be responsible for covering the tight end or running backs. Regardless, the defensive backs are often the smaller but faster players on the defensive side of the ball.

Player substitutions during a football game are unlimited, so players can be interchanged between each play. Depending on the type of play that the offensive coach calls, he may substitute a wide receiver for a running back for a pass play. To counter that substitution, the defensive coach may substitute another defensive back for either a defensive lineman or a linebacker. The only rule regarding players is that the offense is required to have at least five offensive linemen on the field, and a total of seven players have to line up on the line of scrimmage (where the ball is placed). The other four players can line up anywhere behind the line of scrimmage, but they are not permitted to be on the line of scrimmage. Offensive linemen are not eligible to catch the ball or go past the line of scrimmage until the ball itself crosses the line of scrimmage. In contrast, the defensive players are permitted to line up in any location on the field.

In general, football players participate as only offense or defense. The physical demands of the game require maximum intensity on each play that often involves a collision with another player. The intensity of the game has generally eliminated "two-way" players, especially at the higher levels of competition (e.g., college or professional). In youth football, or perhaps even in high school football, some players may have both an offensive position and a defensive position. As discussed earlier, each position on the field has specific responsibilities that create a different physical requirement. The specific distance of movement is also dependent upon the player's position. Offensive and defensive linemen are generally lineup across from one another, which may require a very short distance of movement. Skill position players generally run for greater distances (i.e., 20–40 m) on each play, but they may not experience a physical confrontation on each play. Although the distance that each player moves per play may differ, the intensity for each play is maximal, indicating that the predominant energy systems for all football players is the anaerobic energy system (Hoffman, 2008; Kraemer and Gotshalk, 2000).

The objective of the offense is to score. That can occur in a single play or in a series of plays. The offense has four opportunities, called downs, to move the ball 10 yards. If they are successful, they get another four downs to gain 10 yards. Each time the offense gets 10 yards, it is called a first down. The object of the defense is to stop the offense from gaining 10 yards and either forces them to give the ball up on downs (unsuccessful in four attempts to gain 10 yards) or the offensive decides to "punt" the ball or attempts to kick a field goal on the fourth down. Each group of plays is called a series; thus, a series could be one play, three plays, or if the offensive is successful it may exceed 10–12 plays. The college and professional game comprises four 15-min quarters with a 15-min halftime, while high school games often play 12-min quarters. The number of plays per game will often be determined by offensive coaching philosophy. Some coaches prefer to huddle after each play, letting the quarterback read the defense and make "checks" on the line of scrimmage, while other coaches prefer a "no-huddle" offensive. The no-huddle offense forces the players to play at a much greater pace and will allow them to get more plays in. In an examination of a NCAA Division III football season, an average of 14–15 offensive series per team occurred per game, with an average of four to five plays per series (Hoffman, 2014). This was slightly more than the average number of series reported in National Football League (NFL) games, but less than the number of plays per series (Plisk and Gambetta, 1997). NFL teams run between five and six plays per series. The duration of each play ranges from approximately 2 to 13 s, with the average duration of play lasting approximately 5.5 s in college football (Kraemer and Gotshalk, 2000), but slightly lower (~5.0 s) in the NFL (Plisk and Gambetta, 1997). Iosia and Bishop (2008) examined the top 25 teams in college football. They examined work and rest times, and differences between both run and pass plays. They reported that the average duration of a play was 5.23 ± 1.7 s. Durations of run and pass plays were 4.86 ± 1.4 s and 5.60 ± 1.7 s, respectively. The average duration of rest between plays without extended rest was 36.1 ± 6.7 s, and the average rest time between series was 11.39 ± 4.19 min.

Rest between plays is dependent upon when the referee sets the ball and blows the whistle for the play clock to begin. Once the whistle is blown, each team has a maximum of 25 s to begin the next play. However, as already mentioned, the strategy of some teams may be to line up quickly and snap the ball (i.e., begin the play) with minimal rest to exhaust the opponent or prevent the opponent from substituting rested players. Thus, the rest interval between each play can vary from several seconds to a maximum of 25 s in duration. The average time between plays is reported to be 27–36 s in college and professional football (Iosia and Bishop, 2008; Kraemer and Gotshalk, 2000; Plisk and Gambetta, 1997). However, in teams that play an "up-tempo" style, the time would be less. In addition, the duration of rest is not a true recovery period as during that time a play is called, the players move to the line of scrimmage and make any necessary adjustments. So, the cognitive load is quite heavy during this period of "non-action". Regardless, the ability to determine the average time per play and rest time between plays allows for a more precise understanding of the physiological demands of the game. It also provides important information regarding the development of the anaerobic exercise prescription.

In the past 10 years, technological advancements in the use of global positioning systems (GPS) in sports have provided an ability to examine movement patterns and intensities during competitive football games. One of the first studies using GPS technology to study the game of football was published by Wellman and colleagues (2016). They studied a NCAA Division I football team during the 12-game regular season. The GPS devices were worn by the players in a custom-designed pocket attached to their shoulder pads. The shoulder pads were custom-fit for each individual, thereby minimizing movement of the pads during competition. Only players who participated in 75% of the plays per game were analyzed. Tables 1.1 and 1.2 provide the distance covered on average per game and the average movement intensity of effort for both offensive and defensive positions, respectively. As might be expected, wide receivers and defensive backs covered the greatest distance during the course of a game and performed a greater distance of high intensity and sprint efforts. However, while defensive linemen (both tackles and ends) covered the least distance on defense, running backs covered the lowest distance on offense. However, running backs performed 12.9% of that distance at a high intensity or with greater effort. Defensive players ran 3–4.6 km per game, and about 5.5–16.2% of their distance covered during the games was performed at a high intensity (16.1–23 km·h⁻¹) or sprint (>23 km·h⁻¹) effort. Offensive players ran between 3.1 and 5.5 km per game, and between 3.8% and 17.6% of their distance covered during the games was performed at a high intensity or sprint effort. The percentage of total distance performed at high intensity or greater for all linemen was the lowest of all positions (3.8% and 5.5% for both offensive linemen and defensive tackles, respectively). This is not surprising considering that there is almost immediate contact as soon as the ball is snapped, and these players are rarely able to achieve maximal acceleration before contact.

A subsequent study by Bayliff and colleagues (2019) using GPS technology assessments during a season of competition on NCAA Division I football players reported similar results. In contrast, they reported that the total distance traveled during a game was highest for defensive backs, which was significantly greater than wide receivers ($p = 0.04$) and offensive linemen ($p = 0.01$), but not defensive linemen. In addition, they reported no significant differences in

TABLE 1.1 Distance and Intensity of Effort for Offense

Variable	Offensive Linemen	Tight Ends	Wide Receivers	Running Backs	Quarterbacks
Total distance (m)	3,652 ± 603*	3,574 ± 882*	5,531 ± 997	3,141 ± 686*	3,752 ± 802*
Low intensity (0–10 km·h⁻¹) distance (m)	2,885 ± 664*#&	2,579 ± 664*	3,546 ± 756	2,291 ± 482*	3,662 ± 642#
Moderate intensity (10.1–16 km·h⁻¹) distance (m)	913 ± 148*#&	947 ± 156*#	1,531 ± 341	738 ± 247*	568 ± 148*
High intensity (16.1–23 km·h⁻¹) distance (m)	131 ± 66*#%	337 ± 138*	655 ± 196	303 ± 119*	138 ± 65*#
Sprinting (>23 km·h⁻¹) distance (m)	9 ± 11*#	40 ± 47*	316 ± 163	101 ± 72*	77 ± 46*
Average maximal speed (km·h⁻¹)	23.7 ± 2.8*#&	25.3 ± 7.8*#	31.5 ± 2.2	28.8 ± 2.5*	29.4 ± 8.5

Source: Data adapted from Wellman et al., 2016.

Notes: All data are reported as mean ± SD. * = significantly different ($p < 0.05$) from wide receivers; # = significantly different ($p < 0.05$) from running backs; & = significantly different ($p < 0.05$) from quarterbacks; % = significantly different ($p < 0.05$) from tight ends.

TABLE 1.2 Distance and Intensity of Effort for Defense

Variable	Defensive Tackles	Defensive Ends	Linebackers	Defensive Backs
Total distance (m)	3,013 ± 651*	3,277 ± 815*	4,145 ± 980#&	4,696 ± 1,115
Low intensity (0–10 km·h⁻¹) distance (m)	2,500 ± 457*	2,663 ± 653*	2,989 ± 722#&	3,449 ± 923
Moderate intensity (10.1–16 km·h⁻¹) distance (m)	629 ± 249*	665 ± 224*	913 ± 271#&	926 ± 247
High intensity (16.1–23 km·h⁻¹) distance (m)	159 ± 62*	226 ± 96*	435 ± 165#&	514 ± 156
Sprinting (>23 km·h⁻¹) distance (m)	8 ± 11*	29 ± 24*	197 ± 105#&	247 ± 113
Average maximal speed (km·h⁻¹)	23.5 ± 1.7*	26.1 ± 2.6*#	29.6 ± 1.2#&	31.1 ± 1.9

Source: Data adapted from Wellman et al., 2016.

Notes: All data are reported as mean ± SD. * = significantly different ($p < 0.05$) from defensive backs; # = significantly different ($p < 0.05$) from defensive tackles; & = significantly different ($p < 0.05$) from defensive ends.

distance traveled among wide receivers and both offensive and defensive linemen. As expected, both wide receivers and defensive backs had a higher maximal velocity than offensive linemen. Differences in total distance traveled and maximal velocity between studies may be related to differences in coaching philosophy, as run-oriented teams versus pass-oriented teams would likely have less total distance covered and velocity of movement.

Acute Physiological Response During a Football Game

As discussed earlier, there are a host of logistical issues that have generally limited the ability to research acute physiological changes in an actual football game. In 2001, sport scientists from the College of New Jersey and the University of Connecticut collaborated on the first study to examine the physiological responses during a collegiate football game (Hoffman et al., 2002). The game was the final game of the 2001 season and the head coach of the College of New Jersey, Eric Hamilton, had agreed to allow the research team to set up a mini-laboratory on the sideline. Blood draws were obtained the day before, prior to the game, and immediately following the game. The cooperation was unprecedented, and it was likely facilitated by the primary investigator being a member of the coaching staff, and the fact that our opponent was not strong, the expectation was that we were going to win the game by a significant amount. In addition, Coach Hamilton was a big proponent of the benefits of sport science and he helped facilitate this unique research opportunity. Coach Hamilton was at one time the youngest head coach in the NCAA, when he was named head coach of the College of New Jersey in 1977 at the age of 23. During his 36 years as Head Coach of the NCAA Division III program, among his many great accolades as a football coach and mentor, he continuously promoted sport science and was a huge proponent of the benefits associated with applied sport science research.

During the game, physiological, hormonal, and biochemical changes were examined. Comparisons were made between starters (n = 11) and "red-shirt" freshmen (n = 10; players who were not going to play in order to preserve a year of eligibility). Measures of peak power and peak force were calculated from a vertical jump performed on a force plate, which was set up on the team's sideline. Assessments were performed 10 min prior to the kickoff and at the end of first, second, third, and fourth quarters. In addition, blood samples were obtained 24 and 2.5 h prior to the game and also within 15 min following the contest. Results of the study revealed no significant change in the maximum rate of force development during the game. However, significant decreases were observed in both peak force and peak power at the end of the first quarter of play. These performance variables continued to decline throughout the second quarter. However, both force and power performance returned to baseline levels by the games conclusion. This was likely related to the recovery of players who were substituted for near the game's conclusion. As expected, the game turned into a rout in the second half, which permitted the coaching staff to substitute freely. It is important to acknowledge that in a more closely battled contest, these results may have been quite different.

Hormonal analyses revealed no significant change from baseline in plasma testosterone concentrations, and no difference was noted between starters and red-shirt players. However, a significant elevation in plasma cortisol concentrations was observed in starters, and this elevation was remarkably greater than that in red-shirt players. In addition, plasma myoglobin concentration, a marker of acute muscle damage, was significantly elevated at the conclusion of the game, and it was significantly higher in starters than in red-shirt players. No changes were noted though in plasma creatine kinase concentrations, another marker of muscle damage. The differences observed in the myoglobin and creatine kinase responses were likely related to the timing of the blood draws. Myoglobin is a small molecule and leaks out much quicker from damaged tissue than creatine kinase, which is a much larger molecule. Elevations in plasma myoglobin concentrations will generally peak shortly after exercise, whereas increases in plasma creatine kinase concentrations will generally peak 24–48 h following intense exercise. A post-game blood draw will not provide sufficient time to capture peak elevations in circulating plasma creatine kinase. The results of the Hoffman et al. (2002) study indicated that the rate of force development is maintained, but force and power outputs do decline during the course of a game; however, with strategically managed substitution patterns, force and power performance may be maintained. In addition, hormonal and biochemical responses did suggest increases in muscle damage and stress associated with playing the game.

There is only one additional study known that has examined the acute physiological response to a football game. In contrast to the previous study that was able to examine physiological responses during and immediately after the game, the second investigation examined the players on the day before and after a contest. The investigative team from the University of Connecticut, led by Dr. William Kraemer (2009), examined the biochemical and endocrine response in NCAA Division I football players the day before a game, 18–20 h following the game (e.g., day after game), and 42–44 h after the game (e.g., two days after game). Sixteen starters who played the entire game were compared to 12 players who did not play. Markers of muscle damage (e.g., circulating plasma concentrations of creatine kinase, lactate dehydrogenase, and myoglobin) and the hormones testosterone and cortisol were examined. Significant increases were noted in all markers of muscle damage in the athletes who played in the game. However, no changes were noted in plasma testosterone and cortisol concentrations, and no differences were also noted between players who participated in the game and those who did not in the anabolic and catabolic hormonal responses. These results are consistent with the previous investigation that showed that a game of football may result in an elevation in markers of muscle damage, with minimal disruption to the adrenal–testicular axis.

What Does a Year of Football Consist of?

A year of football consists of several important blocks that are generally referred to as seasons (see Figure 1.1). Figure 1.1 provides an example of a college football year. The part of the year that is focused on preparing for the upcoming competitions is known as the *off-season*. The off-season often represents the end of the previous campaign and the beginning of the next competitive campaign. Oftentimes, new coaching hires occur between the previous campaign and the start of the off-season period, which is the official start of the new campaign. During the off-season, the primary focus of the team is directed at improving the physical ability of the players. There may be some tactical discussions, but for most leagues there is a limit on contact time between coaches and players, which forbids any official football practices. Coaches do have a small window during the off-season period that is often referred to as "spring football or practices" that allow for official football practice, including

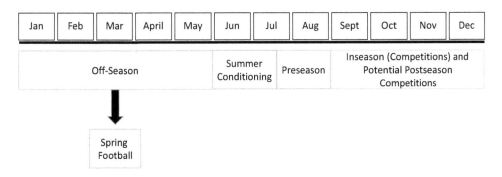

FIGURE 1.1   Example of Seasons in a College Football Player.

full contact. This primarily occurs in NCAA Division I and II football, but not in Division III. At the Division III level, practices are permitted but without pads. In the NFL, there are limited off-season practices that are termed "organized team activities" (OTAs), which was part of the collective bargaining agreement that was negotiated between the NFL and the NFL players association. Teams are allowed to have ten days of OTAs during the off-season to help develop players. The off-season program is focused on increasing strength, power, size, and speed. Chapter 3 will focus primarily on the training programs and their efficacy during this period of time.

Prior to the competitive football season is a period of time that the team begins football practices. This time is known as the "preseason". Depending upon the level of competition, the preseason may be of three to six weeks in duration. Preseason training is quite different today than it was a generation ago. Preseason training was generally associated with high-intensity practice performed twice per day, with limited time for recovery. This period of time, especially the first week of practice, was infamously known as "Hell Week". It was a grueling welcoming to the start of a new football season that was intense, long, and very physical. The incidence of heat illness, including heatstroke leading to player deaths, will be covered in greater detail in Chapter 2. Players generally report to preseason training camp in peak condition, and although strength and conditioning are part of training camp, the primary focus of preseason training is to install the offensive and defensive schemes and have players compete for a starting position. Recent rule changes by the NCAA required its member institutions to limit the number of *two-a-day* practices that take place during the preseason. In addition, rule changes required a gradual increase in equipment used (from helmets only to full practice gear) and reduced the number of practices per day. This appears to have provided players with a sufficient time frame to acclimatize to the heat of summer training camp and enhance their exercise-heat tolerance (Yeargin et al., 2006).

The preseason training camp leads directly to the competitive football season. Training programs developed to maintain strength and power are termed "inseason" training. The competitive football season can last between 10 and 17 weeks, depending upon the league. NCAA Division I football may have a single conference championship game and/or a bowl game. In the past few years, the top four teams are invited to participate in the championship playoffs that may add an additional two games to the competitive season. Lower divisions of NCAA football have a more rigorous playoff format that may add an additional four games to the competitive schedule. Playoff games are considered to be part of the "postseason". The NFL postseason may add an additional three to four postseason games for those teams that reach the Super Bowl (NFL championship game).

Considering the athletes' responsibilities during the preseason, inseason, postseason, and off-season periods, it is clear that the physical stress placed on the football player can be quite significant. However, the ability to quantify or qualify the extent of this stress has been very limited. The next section will provide a review of the existing knowledge that is presently available regarding the stress of playing a competitive football season, including the preseason.

Physiological Demands of a Competitive Football Season

The physiological stress associated with preseason training has been examined in a limited number of studies. One study conducted prior to the change in preseason summer practice rules examined performance and endocrine and biochemical changes during a ten-day, 20-practice training camp in NCAA Division III football players (Hoffman et al., 2004b). The study revealed no significant decrements in strength or power. However, the physicality of football was evident by a significant elevation in serum creatine kinase concentrations at the end of the ten-day training camp. Hormonal analysis indicated no significant change from baseline in plasma testosterone concentrations, but plasma cortisol concentrations were significantly reduced and the testosterone-to-cortisol ratio was elevated. It is likely that cortisol concentrations at the beginning of preseason training camp were elevated, reflecting the anxiety associated with the start of a new football season. Despite elevations in markers of muscle damage, the lack of change in both testosterone and cortisol suggests that highly conditioned athletes were able to withstand the stress of ten-days of two-a-day practices.

A subsequent study examined the physical demands of NCAA Division I college football players during preseason training (DeMartini et al., 2011). Daily practice times averaged 144 ± 13 min per session. The total distance covered during each practice was significantly higher among skill position players (running backs, defensive backs, linebackers, tight ends, and receivers) than linemen (tackles, guards, centers, defensive tackles, and defensive ends) (3.5 ± 0.9 km versus 2.6 ± 0.5 km, respectively). In addition, skill position players were reported to jog ($6.1–12.0$ km·h^{-1}), run ($12.1–16.0$ km·h^{-1}), and sprint (>16 km·h^{-1}) for a significantly longer distance than linemen ($5.1 \pm 1.8\%$ versus $4.1 \pm 1.0\%$, $0.9 \pm 0.0\%$ versus $0.4 \pm 0.5\%$, and $0.8 \pm 0.4\%$ versus $0.1 \pm 0.3\%$, respectively). In addition, no differences were noted between positions in time spent standing or walking (~92–94% of the time). When starting players were compared to nonstarting players, the only significant difference observed during training camp was seen in the time spent standing. Nonstarters spent significantly more time standing ($78.1 \pm 5.6\%$) compared to starters ($74.6 \pm 5.1\%$). No significant differences were noted between skill position players and linemen in average heart rate attained during practice (135 ± 11 beats·min^{-1} versus 136 ± 7 beats·min^{-1}, respectively), but skill position players did reach a significantly higher maximum heart rate (203 ± 8 beats·min^{-1}) than linemen (197 ± 9 beats·min^{-1}).

A couple of other studies have reported on creatine kinase concentrations during preseason training. Ehlers and colleagues (2002), examining 12 NCAA Division I football players during two-a-day practices, reported significant elevations in creatine kinase from 204 ± 67 I·U^{-1} prior at the onset of training camp to $5,125 \pm 5,518$ I·U^{-1} at day 4 of training camp. Creatine kinase concentrations remained elevated at day 7 ($3,370 \pm 3,659$ I·U^{-1}), but it was significantly lower by day 10 ($1,264 \pm 991$ I·U^{-1}). No significant differences were noted in creatine kinase concentrations between day 1 and day 10 of the training camp. The concentrations reported could be considered diagnostic for rhabdomyolysis. Interestingly, these concentrations were much greater than that reported previously (~400 I·U^{-1}) (Hoffman et al., 2004b). The large disparity between these studies is difficult to explain, and it may be related to the athlete's level of conditioning prior to the onset of training camp. Interestingly, a subsequent study by Smoot et al. (2014), who examined 32 NCAA Division I football players during seven days of preseason training, reported creatine kinase levels of $1,300 \pm 2,284$ I·U^{-1} (range: $217–12,067$ I·U^{-1}). Similar to the Ehlers et al. (2002) study, these investigators reported no other symptoms to indicate a diagnosis of rhabdomyolysis, but they suggested that creatine kinase concentrations alone are insufficient to be used as a diagnostic criterion for rhabdomyolysis. Furthermore, the latter group of investigators reported a significant ($p = 0.02$), negative correlation between participation in the number of days of conditioning prior to preseason camp and creatine kinase concentrations. This would partly explain the disparity between the initial study by Hoffman and colleagues (2004b) and the data of both Ehlers et al. (2002) and Smoot et al. (2014). Players in the former study were involved in an organized pretraining camp conditioning program that may have provided a degree of resiliency to the subsequent preseason training camp.

There have been only a handful of studies that have examined the physiological changes in football players during the competitive or inseason period. The first group of investigators to examine competitive football players during the season were the sport scientists from the College of New Jersey (Hoffman et al., 2005b). This investigation compared the biochemical and hormonal responses in starters and nonstarters during a NCAA Division III football season. The investigators reported minimal disruption to the adrenal–testicular axis (e.g., no significant changes in resting testosterone or cortisol concentrations outside of that seen during training camp). Furthermore, the significant elevations observed in creatine kinase concentrations at the end of training camp returned to baseline levels by the first month of the season and remained at these levels throughout the remainder of the season in both starters and nonstarters. This response pattern suggested a degree of desensitization of skeletal muscle to the repeated traumas occurring during the season. This phenomenon has been termed "contact adaptation" (Hoffman et al., 2005b). This has subsequently been supported by other investigative teams (Kraemer et al., 2013), who reported a similar response pattern in NCAA Division I football players. Contact adaptation observed in football players is considered a physiological adaptation to a season of competition providing a mechanism for the player to withstand the physical punishment associated with the game of football (Hoffman, 2008).

Stone and colleagues (2019) followed 20 NCAA Division I football players from the end of the off-season conditioning period until the completion of the competitive season. The athletes were separated into starters (n = 11; players who participated between 20 and 40 repetitions per game) and nonstarters (n = 9). The initial blood draw was obtained before the summer conditioning program; a second blood draw was obtained at the end of the summer conditioning program but before preseason training. There was no football practice, nor physical contact between the first two blood draws. The third blood draw was obtained following preseason training; the fourth and eighth blood draws were obtained during the competitive season, with no more than 28 days between each blood draw. All blood draws were obtained following an 8-h fast, while the inseason blood draws were obtained approximately 48 h following the previous game. Results indicated that starters had higher testosterone concentrations than nonstarters, and that this remained consistent throughout the competitive season. Cortisol concentrations were reported to remain relatively unchanged during all testing periods in nonstarters. However, a small to moderate increase from baseline was observed in starters during the inseason blood draws (fourth and fifth testing points). Interestingly, cortisol concentrations were likely lower at the end of preseason training camp in starters compared to nonstarters, but no changes were observed relative to baseline in either group of players. Creatine kinase concentrations were significantly higher than baseline concentrations at every time point measured, and starters were observed to have higher creatine kinase concentrations than nonstarters at all testing points except the first and eighth testing points. The creatine kinase response did not support the previously discussed contact adaptation phenomenon.

Physiological adaptation during the competitive season also appears to involve muscle oxygen kinetics and recovery (Hoffman et al., 2004c). In a study of NCAA Division III football players, 30-s Wingate anaerobic power tests were performed throughout the season. In addition, immediately after each Wingate test muscle oxygenation, deoxygenation and reoxygenation were measured using near-infrared spectroscopy (NIRS). Testing was initiated at the onset of training camp and then every four weeks until the end of the regular season. A total of four tests were conducted. Results showed a significant reduction in the magnitude of muscle deoxygenation and a significant faster time for reoxygenation. This adaptation appeared to occur without any significant change in peak power, mean power, rate of fatigue, and total work performed during the monthly assessments. Players were able to maintain power performance and fatigue rate throughout the competitive season. In addition, their ability to reoxygenate muscle appeared to have improved.

What Is the Ability of Football Players to Maintain Strength During the Competitive Season?

The primary goal of an inseason strength and conditioning program is to maintain the performance gains that were achieved during the previous off-season conditioning program. There have been several studies examining the effect of an inseason training program on strength and power performance. When an inseason maintenance program is employed, football players appear to be able to maintain both upper and lower body strength during the competitive season (Hoffman and Kang, 2003). Maintenance of strength appears to be accomplished while using a two-day per week maintenance program, with loads equating to 80% of the athletes maximal strength (1RM) in each core exercise (i.e., bench press, squat, power cleans, and push press). Interestingly, when training intensity is at or greater than 80% of the 1RM, the ability to stimulate strength improvements is significantly greater than when training intensity is below 80%, especially in first-year players (Hoffman and Kang, 2003). It is possible that the accumulated fatigue occurring in players who have greater playing time limits the extent of muscle adaptation during the season.

Examination of the Use of GPS Technology to Assess Player Load/Intensity in Football

As discussed earlier, the use of GPS technology has provided a noninvasive approach to analyze the stress of games and a season of competition. Although GPS technology is used among various teams and leagues, the number of scientific publications discussing their findings is limited. Recently, Wellman and colleagues (2019) reported on player load comparisons between preseason and inseason practice and games. Player load, which is used synonymously with training load, was determined by combined triaxial accelerometer data and expressed as the square root of the sum of the squared instantaneous rates of change in acceleration in each of the three planes and divided by 100. In addition, they performed position comparisons. The research team observed significant differences in player load between preseason and inseason practices in NCAA Division I football players. Preseason practices were significantly more intense (3,087 arbitrary units [au]) than inseason practices (1,524 au). This was thought to be at least partly related to the greater average practice duration of the preseason practices (2.09 h) compared to the inseason practices (1.47 h). These results also emphasize the importance for football players to report to preseason training camp in a high level of condition.

Cardiovascular Profile of Football Players

A number of studies have examined the cardiovascular profile of football players at various levels of competition (Crouse et al., 2016; Edenfield et al., 2019; Kim et al., 2018; Lin et al., 2016; Tucker et al., 2009; Uberoi et al., 2013; Weiner et al., 2013). In a cross-sectional study of more than 500 active, veteran NFL players from 12 teams, Tucker and colleagues (2009) reported that professional football players are at a higher risk for hypertension than age-matched control men. Both systolic and diastolic blood pressure measurements were significantly greater than that seen in the age-matched controls. However, these levels were still within normal range. The larger blood pressure response was likely related to the greater height and weight in the NFL player population. The NFL players had a significantly greater body mass index (BMI) than the age-matched controls. No other differences were noted between the two populations in any other cardiovascular disease risk factor (e.g., blood lipids). The authors concluded that the NFL players, characterized by a larger body size and more intense physical activity, had a cardiovascular risk profile that was similar to the general population. Difference in blood pressure was noted between positions, with NFL linemen having higher blood pressure readings than the skill position players. This is a finding that has been repeated in numerous investigations examining other levels of competition. Uberoi and colleagues (2013) examined 85 NCAA Division I football players during their preparticipation exam. They compared linemen, mobility/power players (e.g., linebackers and fullbacks), and skill position players on a variety of cardiovascular measures. The results of their study indicated that linemen had a greater heart mass than the other positions, even after adjustment and correction for body surface area. Furthermore, left ventricular (LV) end-systolic volume, LV diastolic volume, and LV ejection fraction were not significantly different between positions after adjusting for body surface area. ECG measures indicated that QRS duration was correlated with LV mass. Table 1.3 compares cardiovascular dimensions between different positions.

The effect of a season of competition on cardiovascular parameters has been examined in a limited number of studies. Weiner and colleagues (2013) reported that during preseason assessments, linemen had significantly higher systolic (119 ± 8 versus 113 ± 8 mmHg) and diastolic blood pressure (66 ± 8 versus 62 ± 9 mmHg) than skill position players, respectively. By the end of the season, blood pressure in the linemen was significantly elevated (131 ± 11 mmHg), which was considered to be prehypertensive. The investigators also examined changes in echocardiographic measures and reported significant differences in left ventricular mass between linemen (228 ± 27 g) and skill position (214 ± 25 g) players, which became significantly elevated during the season for all players. These differences were still evident when examined relative to body size. At

TABLE 1.3 Positional Comparison of Cardiovascular Dimensions

Variable	Linemen (n = 34)	Mobility/Power (n = 13)	Skill Position (n = 38)
LVM (g)*	220 ± 40	175 ± 29	154 ± 24
LVM adjusted for BSA (g·m^{-1})*	86 ± 15	77 ± 12	72 ± 9
LVED diameter (mm)*	57 ± 5	53 ± 4	51 ± 4
LVED diameter adjusted for BSA (mm·m^{-1})	22 ± 2	23 ± 2	24 ± 2
LVES diameter (mm)*	35 ± 6	34 ± 3	32 ± 4
LVES diameter adjusted for BSA (mm·m^{-1})	14 ± 3	15 ± 2	15 ± 2
LV posterior wall thickness (mm)*	10.3 ± 1.2	9.1 ± 1.1	8.8 ± 1.1
Intraventricular septal thickness (mm)*	9.5 ± 1.5	8.9 ± 1.7	8.2 ± 0.9
LVEF (%)	62 ± 8	61 ± 7	61 ± 6

Source: Data from Uberoi et al., 2013.

Notes: Linemen include both offensive and defensive; mobility/power includes both linebackers and fullbacks; and skill position includes all remaining players. LVM = left ventricular mass; BSA = body surface area; LVED = left ventricular end-diastolic; LVES = left ventricular end-systolic; LVEF = left ventricular ejection fraction; * = significant difference between players.

postseason, 32% of the players examined were demonstrated to have LV hypertrophy. No differences were noted in the appearance of LV hypertrophy between linemen and skill position players. However, the geometric pattern of LV hypertrophy did differ by position. Concentric LV hypertrophy was the dominant pattern among linemen (83%), but it was present in only 8% of skill position players. In addition, changes in LV mass were significantly associated with changes in systolic blood pressure. Weiner and colleagues (2013) suggested that the changes in cardiovascular measures, especially among the linemen, required a greater surveillance and potential intervention to improve later-life cardiovascular health outcomes in these athletes. Cardiovascular risk for these athletes during their post-career days will be discussed in greater detail in Chapter 7.

Other investigators have also raised concern regarding cardiovascular health in football players (Crouse et al., 2016; Kim et al., 2018; Lin et al., 2016). Although Crouse and colleagues (2016) reported that 78% of the first-year NCAA Division I football players (n = 80) were overweight or obese by body mass index, they did acknowledge that 72% of those athletes had a body composition level that was below 20% body fat. The vast majority of athletes were not overfat, and the investigators emphasized the lack of sensitivity of population-based body mass index standards to football athletes as a measure of obesity. Recently, Edenfield et al. (2019) have indicated that nonathlete norms do not apply to various echocardiographic data such as LV end-diastolic diameter (LVEDD) and intraventricular septal diameter (IVSD) values in a college football population. They suggested that body surface area (BSA) has the strongest association with LVEDD and IVSD values and that the values in collegiate football players that approach the upper limits of nonathlete norms should be interpreted in the context of BSA.

Limited research has compared cardiovascular changes among football players of different age groups. Kim and colleagues (2018) compared the cardiovascular response of high school and college football players. They reported that the transition from high school to college represented an important physiological point where cardiovascular adaptation manifested differently. While both high school and college players demonstrated similar and significant increases in LV mass index and wall thickness during the competitive season, differences were reported in LV geometric remodeling patterns. Although there was no difference in the change in LV diameter relative to body size between high school and collegiate players, there were significantly higher rates of concentric LV hypertrophy observed among college (24%) versus high school players (11%). LV systolic function, as assessed by ejection fraction and global longitudinal strain, was unchanged among the high school players, but it showed a nonsignificant trend toward a decline among the college athletes. Differences in diastolic function were also noted. Early filling rate (E′) significantly declined during the season among college players, but it was unchanged in the high school players. These differences were significantly different between the two age groups. Similar responses were also noted for vascular function. High school football players experienced stable vascular compliance during the competitive season, while college players demonstrated arterial stiffening as evidenced by significant increases in pulse wave velocity at the end of the competitive season. The differences between the groups were also significant. The results of this study highlighted differential cardiovascular remodeling patterns in high school and college football players. The long-term cardiovascular health implications of these findings are not well understood. However, further research on differences in cardiovascular remodeling patterns appears warranted.

A recent study examined heart rate variability (HRV) in Division I college players during four weeks of spring football practices (Flatt et al., 2018). HRV is thought to reflect autonomic modulation of the heart. Vagally mediated HRV is a marker of homeostasis, reflecting cardiovascular recovery following exercise (Stanley et al., 2013). A return to vagal HR following exercise would be considered to be an indicator of complete recovery. This study examined the time-domain vagal HRV index of the natural logarithm of the root mean square of successive RR intervals (lnRMSSD) to provide insight into recovery. Results demonstrated that daily lnRMSSD responses to a football training session differed by position. Twenty hours after a practice session, linemen showed substantial reductions from baseline in comparison to skill position players who recovered to within or near baseline values. Linemen do appear to be at greater risk for inadequate recovery than skill position players, potentially making them susceptible to autonomic nervous system imbalance during more intense practice sessions.

Summary

Research examining the physiological response to a competitive football game is very limited. It does appear that with proper manipulation of substitution patterns during a game, the force and power performance can be maintained. There are several physiological adaptations noted in football players during the season, including a greater desensitization to physical contact. This evidence provides support for an increased resiliency among the players, and perhaps it is a potential inherent mechanism for injury prevention. Evidence was also presented that reported on position-specific demands that differ, especially among linemen and skill position players.

2

ENVIRONMENTAL CONCERNS OF PLAYING AMERICAN FOOTBALL

Introduction

Football is one of the few sports in the world whose players may experience all facets of environmental extremes in a single season. Training camp for all players, at all levels, begins in the middle of the summer. The risk for heat illness is significant, and coaches need to be cognizant of the risk associated with exercise in the heat and adjust practices accordingly. As training camp concludes, the season that began in the summer continues into the fall. However, for football players on the northeastern quadrant of the United States, where winter comes quickly and briskly, the temperature begins to drop toward the end of the season and the risk for cold-related injuries becomes more significant. In addition, players who generally play at a destination that is near sea level may be required to travel to a game at altitude. For example, if the New England Patriots, who practice in Massachusetts at an elevation of 43 m, travel to play the Denver Broncos, whose elevation is 1,609 m ("the mile high city"), what type of physiological stress does that impose on the Patriot players compared to the Denver Broncos? Are the Patriots at a physiological disadvantage? What about the New York Jets flying to play the San Francisco 49ers for a Monday night game. Does the 3-h time difference impact the physiology of the players? What about the NFL players who fly to Great Britain to play on a yearly basis? Does the multiple time zone changes affect performance? These environmental extremes are the focus of this chapter. Playing in the heat, cold, and at altitude and crossing multiple time zones create physiological challenges that if not acknowledged can place the athlete at risk, with possible lethal consequences.

To better understand the impact of these environmental extremes on football performance, it becomes imperative to provide a brief overview of environmental stress.

The Effect of Heat on Football Performance

Physical activity results in a greater need for energy that can result in an increase in metabolic rate 5–15 times higher than that seen at rest (Hoffman, 2014). This higher metabolic rate creates a large heat production that needs to be dissipated for thermal homeostasis to be maintained. This places a large burden on the thermoregulatory system to defend the body's core temperature. When an athlete begins to exercise in the heat, the thermoregulatory system is further stressed. The extent of the physiological stress depends on several factors, including the athlete's heat acclimatization, level of physical fitness, and hydration state. These factors can affect the athlete's ability to perform. In addition, exercising in the heat may pose a significant risk to the health and well-being of the athlete.

The primary goal of the body's thermoregulatory system is to remove the heat from the body. An increase in body temperature is called hyperthermia (elevated body temperature). Changes in core temperature are monitored by the hypothalamus, which determines when an imbalance in temperature homeostasis has occurred, and if so activates a mechanism of action to return core temperature to normal levels. This results in sweat gland activation to stimulate sweat production, and the smooth muscle in the arterioles of the skin are relaxed to allow for vasodilation and an increase in blood flow to the periphery by diverting blood flow from internal organs to the skin to expedite heat dissipation (Hoffman, 2014).

If the body is unable to maintain temperature homeostasis, the risk for the athlete to suffer a heat illness increases. This risk will be highlighted and discussed in the next section in more detail. However, to understand the potential risk for the football player, it is important to understand how the body dissipates heat to the environment. Heat is dissipated through both evaporative and nonevaporative means. Evaporative heat loss involves evaporation of water (the result of sweating) from the body. Evaporation accounts for approximately 85–90% of the heat dissipation during exercise in a hot, dry environment (Adams et al., 1975). Keep in mind that when the air is dry, it is not filled with moisture. A desert environment would be an example of a hot, dry environment. So the water droplets on the skin from the athlete's perspiration are easily evaporated into the air. However, in a hot and wet environment, which may be experienced by athletes exercising by a large body of water (i.e., ocean), the moisture in the air limits evaporation. Moisture is measured as humidity. As the moisture in the air increases, evaporative heat loss is reduced and a greater amount of heat is stored in the body. During humid conditions (hot and wet), the skin becomes hot and reddish in color, which represents the increased blood that has been diverted to the periphery. The body relies more on nonevaporative mechanisms to dissipate heat. Nonevaporative heat loss is the result of the combined effects of conduction, radiation, and convection. Conduction is heat exchange between two solid surfaces that are in direct contact. The rate of conductance depends on the temperature difference between the two surfaces. Conduction may have limited value during exercise in the heat because of the limited surface area that is in direct contact with the ground. It accounts for less than 2% of heat loss in most situations (Armstrong, 2000). Radiation is the transfer of energy waves that are emitted by one object and absorbed by another (Armstrong, 2000). Convection is heat exchange that occurs between a surface and a fluid medium. Both air and body fluids can dissipate heat through convective means. As mentioned previously, evaporative heat loss is severely reduced during exercise in a hot, wet environment. Thus, the body relies more on radiation and convection to dissipate heat under these conditions.

Unlike evaporative cooling, which always dissipates heat, the ability of radiation and convection to reduce body heat is dependent on ambient temperature. If skin temperature is greater than ambient temperature, then heat would leave the body. However, if skin temperature is less than ambient temperature, heat would likely be added to the body. During conditions in which both ambient temperature and humidity are high, the ability to dissipate heat through either evaporative or nonevaporative mechanisms becomes limited. In such conditions, the athlete will have difficulty dissipating body heat and will be at an increased risk for heat illness.

The use of a uniform, specifically a football uniform, can further exacerbate the strain of performing in the heat. The uniform ensemble (helmet, shoulder pads, girdle, pants, jersey) may result in an *uncompensable heat stress* that minimizes evaporative cooling. Uncompensable heat stress exists when the evaporative cooling requirements exceed the environment's cooling capacity (Givoni and Goldman, 1972). A system of evaluating the insulating effect of clothing has been developed for understanding the effect various layers of clothing has on the ability to gain or lose heat. The unit used for measuring clothing insulation is *Clo* and is reported as $m^2 \cdot K \cdot W^{-1}$ (square meter Kelvin per watt) (1 Clo = 0.155 as $m^2 \cdot K \cdot W^{-1}$). A naked person has a Clo value of 0.0 and a person wearing a typical business suit would have Clo value of 1.0. The Clo value is calculated by summing the Clo values of all clothing layers. As might be expected, evaporative heat transfer is affected by the thickness of the clothing ensemble. The moisture permeability index (*im*) provides a value that determines the permeability of moisture that the ambient air can evaporate (Havenith et al., 1999). An im of 0 represents an impermeable layer of clothing, whereas an im of 1 indicates all of the moisture can be evaporated. A typical im value for most permeable clothing ensembles in "still air" is about 0.5.

The equipment worn by a football player during a game has been reported to range from 1.15 to 1.50 Clo and the permeability index ranged from 0.37 to 0.40 im (McCullough and Kenney, 2003). Dr. Larry Armstrong and colleagues (2010) examined two football uniform ensembles; a partial uniform ensemble that included compression shorts, socks, shoes, gloves, t-shirt, jersey, pants with knee, and thigh pads, while the full uniform included everything previously mentioned plus the shoulder pads and helmet. A control condition was used in which participants wore compression shorts, athletic shorts, socks, and shoes only. This was a laboratory study in which participants were required to walk 80 min on a treadmill followed by performing box lifts in a hot environment (33°C, 48–49% relative humidity). The investigators reported that performance in the full uniform reduced time to exhaustion and increased the rate of core temperature elevation compared to the other uniform ensembles. These results were similar to a previous study examining offensive linemen simulating football-specific drills in various uniform ensembles, and reported that the addition of shoulder pads to the helmet resulted in a significant increase in core temperature, by about 0.3°C (Hitchcock et al., 2007). Clearly, changing the uniform ensemble can ease the physiological strain on the athlete.

It is important that decisions regarding uniform ensembles are based on specific environmental conditions. Increases in both core and skin temperatures can occur in various uniform ensembles without the athlete being able to perceive the difference in physiological strain (Johnson et al., 2010). Thus, it is important not to rely solely on the athlete's perception but to use a standardized approach in deciding what uniform ensemble is appropriate for practice. Interestingly, greater core temperatures in football players have also been reported to be associated with greater aggression and with the potential for greater aggressive penalties (Craig et al., 2016),

Can Heat Stress Be Monitored?

To maximize the safety of athletes, an ability to quantify the strain of the thermal environment through the development of an index can be used to minimize heat-related injuries and make appropriate adjustments to training schedules. A heat stress index integrates the effects of the basic parameters on a thermal environment that vary with the thermal strain experienced by an athlete (Hoffman, 2014). There have been a number of heat stress indices that have been developed. Some of them though may be too complicated to be used by personnel in the field to be effective.

One of the more accepted indices is the wet bulb globe temperature (WBGT). WBGT is a widely used heat stress index that can be measured at the site of activity and used to indicate the level of environmental stress (Armstrong, 2000). The WBGT can quantify perceived heat stress imposed through all four heat exchange pathways. It consists of a dry bulb temperature (measuring ambient air temperature), a wet bulb temperature (dry bulb thermometer measured under a water-saturated cloth wick), and a black globe temperature (dry bulb thermometer placed inside a black metal sphere). It provides both ambient temperature and relative humidity at the site of activity. The black globe temperature provides a measure of the full absorbance of radiation and constant exposed surface area, regardless of location of radiative heat source. The importance of this apparatus compared to ambient temperature alone is that ambient temperature (e.g., dry bulb temperature) accounts for only 10% of the heat stress index, whereas the wet bulb temperature (indication of relative humidity) accounts for 70% of the heat stress index (Yaglou and Minard, 1957). The WBGT index is as follows:

WBGT = (0.7 temperature wet bulb) + (0.2 temperature black globe) + (0.1 temperature dry bulb)

In the absence of a significant radiant load, the equation can be

WBGT = (0.7 temperature wet bulb) + (0.3 temperature dry bulb)

A WBGT index above 82°F (28°C) places the athlete at a very high risk for heat illness. A WBGT index between 73°F and 82°F (23–28°C) places the athlete at a high risk for heat illness. A WBGT index between 64°F and 73°F (18–23°C) places the athlete at a moderate risk, and a WBGT index below 64°F (18°C) is considered a low risk for heat illness. Although a heat stress index of 63°F (17°C) is considered a low risk for heat illness, there is no guarantee that the athlete will not experience heat exhaustion or exertional heatstroke. A number of different factors (e.g., sleep deprivation, hydration status, and diet) may interact to increase the individual's risk of heat illness, even at a relatively low heat stress index (Epstein, 1990).

What Is the Risk of Playing Football in the Heat?

There are several types of heat illnesses commonly seen among athletes: *heat cramps*, *heat exhaustion*, *exertional heatstroke*, and *heat syncope*. Although there is some thought that these heat illnesses exist in a continuum, an athlete may exhibit symptoms of any of these heat illnesses without expressing symptoms of any other (Armstrong and Maresh, 1993). The incidence of any of these heat illnesses is reduced when the athlete becomes acclimatized to the heat (Armstrong and Maresh, 1991). Heat cramps are associated with painful contractions within exercising muscles. They are believed to be the result of a large loss of electrolytes (Na^+ and Cl^-) in sweat and/or the replacement of sweat loss with dilute fluid, pure water, or both (Armstrong, 2000). Heat exhaustion is the most common form of heat illness. It is considered a volume depletion issue that occurs when cardiac output is reduced. Decreases in cardiac output occur from both the shunting of blood from the body's core to its periphery (skin) to enhance cooling and the loss of fluid via perspiration. At some point, the cardiovascular system becomes unable to maintain the demands of exercising muscle while shunting blood to peripheral tissues, and exercise will not be able to continue. Symptoms of heat exhaustion include various combinations of nausea, vomiting, irritability, headache, anxiety, diarrhea, chills, piloerection, hyperventilation, tachycardia, hypotension, and heat sensations in the head and upper torso (Armstrong, 2000). Athletes may also feel dizzy and can faint (heat syncope). Rectal temperature is usually less than 40°C. The signs and symptoms of heat exhaustion may be quite variable and may differ under different exercise-heat scenarios (Armstrong and Maresh, 1993).

Unlike heat exhaustion, in which the athlete's ability to continue to exercise is severely limited, heatstroke can threaten the life of the athlete. Generally, it is seen in a highly motivated athlete who is pushing himself past a point of comfort. Core temperature continues to elevate and cellular damage is seen. During heatstroke, the ability of the body's cooling mechanism is absent. An athlete suffering from heatstroke will have hot, dry skin. In addition, another characteristic associated with heatstroke is bizarre behavior. A person who has exertional heatstroke may be disoriented with complete loss of mental acuity.

One of the most infamous incidents of exertional heatstroke leading to an unfortunate death occurred on August 1, 2001, when Korey Stringer, an All-Pro offensive tackle with the Minnesota Vikings, became the first and to date only National Football League (NFL) player to die of heatstroke during practice. It created a tremendous awareness of the dangers of heatstroke and an opportunity to study the risks and predisposing factors associated with exertional heatstroke. As a result of Korey Stringer's death, the NFL with the Stringer family helped create the Korey Stringer Institute, which is led by Dr. Douglas Casa at the University of Connecticut. Dr. Casa is one of the leading scientists in the world studying heat illness in athletes. He has spent his professional career examining ways to prevent heat illness and educate coaches, trainers, and athletes on methods to reduce the risk associated with exercising in the heat. Dr. Andrew Grundstein, along with Dr. Casa and three other investigators, published a "case study" on the Korey Stringer incident (Grundstein et al., 2017). From court records, the practices preceding the fatal incident were detailed:

> On the first day of training camp in Mankato, MN (July 30, 2001), Stringer participated in morning and afternoon training sessions. He struggled during the afternoon practice. After 45 min, he vomited twice and was brought to an on-field trailer by a Minnesota Viking staff member. A physician employed by the Minnesota Vikings reported that Stringer experienced an episode of heat exhaustion. Stringer returned the next day (July 31, 2001) and participated in high-intensity practice drills in full pads (helmet, shoulder pads, jersey, girdle pads, pants) on an unusually hot and humid morning. Stringer continued to train despite vomiting, sweating profusely, and showing signs of distress. Eyewitness accounts indicated that on several occasions during training, he fell to his knees or to the ground. Upon completing practice at around 11:15 a.m., he collapsed on the practice field. An ambulance arrived at 12:08 p.m. but court documents indicate that no cooling occurred during transport. Medical treatment began upon arrival at the hospital at 12:24 p.m. where his core temperature was 42.67°C. Stringer ultimately died from heat stroke at 1:50 a.m. on August 1, 2001.

The incident was shocking to the world of professional football and led to a number of changes. However, most importantly, it directed a spotlight on the issue of exertional heatstroke. Although Korey Stringer was the first and only NFL player to die from heatstroke, this has been an issue for football for 70 years.

The number of heatstroke deaths in football by decade can be observed in Figure 2.1. The highest amount of deaths were seen in the 1960s and 1970s (35 and 31 deaths per decade, respectively) (Kucera et al., 2017). These numbers began to decline in the 1980s and 1990s (14 and 16 deaths, respectively), but began an uptick again in the new millennium. In the 1970s, the concept of water breaks was used as a "reward" for hard work. It was not an expected occurrence. In fact, many coaches withheld water as a punishment or to "toughen up" their athletes. The education of coaches regarding the importance of water and the risk of dehydration

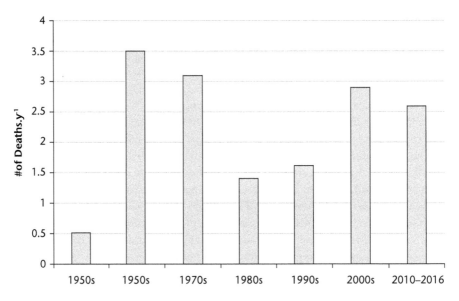

FIGURE 2.1 Relative Heatstroke Deaths per Decade in Football.

Source: Data adapted from Kucera et al., 2017.

changed the way coaches behaved. By the 1980s, NFL training camps had water stations available at every part of the field where players practiced. Staying hydrated was never an issue for players who understood the importance of hydrating. The results of these behavioral changes are clearly seen in Figure 2.1. The reasons for the uptick in heatstroke deaths in the new millennial are not clear, but they likely range from lack of education to simple incompetence.

From 2009 through 2015, there were 174 heat illness injuries that were recorded in National Collegiate Athlete Association (NCAA) football programs (Yeargin et al., 2019), while 216 heat illness injuries were recorded in high school football programs during 2012–2017 (Kerr et al., 2019). This represented 75% and 72%, respectively, of all heat illness injuries across all sports reported in the country. Clearly, the sport of football presents the greatest risk for heat illness, and this is related to the large number of participants per team, the time of the year it is played, practice times, and insufficient monitoring of the athletes. The most common heat illness reported among college football players was heat cramps (43.1%), followed by heat exhaustion (28.7%) (Yeargin et al., 2019). In this specific study, dehydration alone was considered as a heat illness by itself and accounted for 24.7% of the heat illnesses. Of the schools participating in this study, only one case of exertional heatstroke was reported in college football during this time period. However, it was not clear whether this time period included off-season conditioning programs that also may have experienced cases of heatstroke. In the study of high school athletes, heat exhaustion was reported in 61.1% of the football players diagnosed with a heat illness, while 20.4% of these players suffered heat cramps (Kerr et al., 2019). In that same study, 9.3% of the football players had a heat syncope episode and 1.4% of the football players were diagnosed with heatstroke. Nearly 8% of the heat illnesses reported were unknown.

Meteorological conditions play an important role in the risk for heat illness. Although heatstrokes have been reported in a wide range of meteorological conditions, the median conditions that are associated with exertional heatstroke are hot and humid, with a WBGT greater than 30°C (Grundstein et al., 2018). When examining different geographical regions of the United

TABLE 2.1 Guidelines for Modification for Practice Sessions and Competition in the Heat Using WBGT

WBGT		Competition	Practice for Fit, Acclimated Athletes
°F	°C		
≤ 50.0	≤ 10.0	Generally safe	Normal practice
50.1–65.0	10.1–18.3	Generally safe	Normal practice
65.1–72.0	18.4–22.2	Risk of exertional heat illnesses increase, high-risk individuals should be monitored	Normal practice
72.1–78.0	22.3–25.6	Risk for all players is increased	Normal practice, monitor fluid intake
78.1–82.0	25.7–27.8	Risk for all players is high, regardless of fitness level	Normal practice, monitor fluid intake
82.1–86.0	27.9–30.0	Risk for unfit, unacclimatized players is high	Plan intense or prolonged practice with discretion, monitor at-risk athletes
86.1–90.0	30.1–32.2	Risk is very high, consider cancelling event	Limit intense exercise and total daily exposure to heat and humidity, watch for early signs and symptoms
≥ 90.1	≥ 32.3		Cancel practice, uncompensable heat stress exists for all athletes

Source: Adapted from Armstrong et al., 2007.

States, several areas of the country have been identified as having a greater risk for heat illness, specifically exertional heatstroke. The maximum WBGTs ranged between 28°C and 32.0°C, with many of the greatest values exceeding 32°C in the southern part of the United States (Grundstein et al., 2018). To reduce the risk for heat illnesses, the American College of Sports Medicine (ACSM) has suggested that adjustments in practice times, duration, water breaks, or cancellation be implemented (Armstrong et al., 2007). Table 2.1 provides an overview of the guidelines suggested by the ACSM on competition and practice in the heat. For football programs from the southern part of the United States or other areas with constant heat stress indices, practice schedules, game times, and other modifications should become part of the norm. For programs in more temperate environments, sudden weather changes should be monitored and necessary adjustments implemented to reduce risk.

In addition to environmental considerations, there are several other predisposing factors that may increase a football player's risk for heat illness, especially exertional heatstroke. These risk factors can be considered physiological, organizational, and treatment (Minard, 1961). Physiological individual limitations include any underlying illness, level of physical fitness, hydration status, sleep pattern, obesity, and acclimatization status. Organizational factors focus on practice plans: Do the requirements of practice meet the fitness level of the players; does work/rest cycles need to be adjusted; are water stations and fluid easily available; is a hydration plan in place; and does practice need to be adjusted to avoid practicing at the hottest times of the day? Finally, is there a plan in place to rapidly cool the athletes; and is the training staff or coaching staff familiar with all procedures to diagnose and treat any player exhibiting signs and symptoms of a heat illness?

What Is the Importance of Heat Acclimatization?

In a four-year study examining exertional heat illness rates in college football players, the risk of heat illness was most prevalent during the initial 14 days of preseason practice (Cooper et al., 2016). As a result of the greater risk for heat illness during the initial days of football practice, the NCAA and high school football associations created specific practice guidelines to help acclimatize football players to the heat and reduce the risk for heat injury (see Table 2.2). Heat acclimatization is a process that increases the tolerance of a person to a hot environment. There are a number of physiological adaptations that improve the thermoregulatory function of the body. When such adaptation occurs in a naturally hot environment, it is termed acclimatization. Acclimation is the term used when it occurs artificially such as in an environmental chamber; however, the physiological effects are the same. Acclimatization occurs after repeated exposures to a heat stress that is sufficient to raise core body temperature and bring about moderate to profuse sweating (Wenger, 1988). Heat acclimatization appears to occur in two stages. The initial stage, seen after only a few days of heat exposure, is associated with a reduction in cardiovascular strain (e.g., reduced heart rate), increase in plasma volume, increase in exercise tolerance, and decreases in both core temperature and perceived levels of exertion (Armstrong and Maresh, 1991; Wenger, 1988). As the duration of heat exposure is prolonged (up to 14 days), further adaptations may

TABLE 2.2 Comparison of NCAA and High School Acclimatization Policies

	NCAA	High School
Length of acclimatization period	Five-day acclimatization period	14-day acclimatization period
Equipment allowed during acclimatization	• Days 1 and 2 only helmets • Days 3 + 4 only helmets and shoulder pads • Day 5 full equipment	• Days 1 and 2 only helmets • Days 3–5 only helmets and shoulder pads • Day 6+ full equipment
Single practice days	Practice time should not exceed 3 h	• Practice time should not exceed 3 h • A 1-h walkthrough is allowed if 3 h separated by at least 3 h
Double practice days	• May have a 1-h testing session and a 2-h practice on one of the five days • 3 h of recovery must separate the two sessions	• Only on days 6+ • Must be followed by a single-practice day • Must be separated by 3 h of rest • Neither practice should be longer than 3 h • Total practice time should not be longer than 5 h • Double-practice days
Missed day policy	All athletes must complete the heat acclimatization period regardless of arrival to preseason practice	Days that athletes do not practice, either individually or team-wide, do not count to the 14 days
Drills allowed during practice		• Football may use tackling dummies and blocking sleds on days 3+ • Live contact drills may begin on day 6

Source: Adapted from the Korey Stringer Institute, University of Connecticut Neag School of Education, www.ksi.uconn.edu

be observed. These include increases in sweat rate and sweat sensitivity (i.e., sweat loss expressed for degree rise of core body temperature), as well as a decrease in electrolyte losses in both sweat and urine (Armstrong and Maresh, 1991; Wenger, 1988).

In one of the first investigations to examine the effectiveness of the NCAA acclimatization policy, Yeargin and colleagues (2006) monitored football players during days 1–8 of preseason practice. The meteorological conditions during the eight-day study ranged from warm–humid to hot–humid and practice intensities increased over the duration of the study. Physiological measures indicated that heart rate differed significantly within and across days, but no changes were noted in core temperatures at the end of practice. However, the increasing practice intensity and difference in heat strain between practices made it very difficult to clearly see the benefits of the heat acclimatization protocol. In a retrospective study, Kerr and colleagues (2019) examined the effectiveness of heat acclimation in high school football for over 12 years and reported that the high school athletic association's mandated heat acclimatization guidelines were associated with a 55% reduction in the incidence of exertional heat illness. This clearly indicated the effectiveness of the gradual introduction of players to football practices for reducing heat illness.

Are Linemen at Greater Risk Than Skill Position Players for Exertional Heat Illness?

One of the predisposing factors associated with greater risk of heat illness is obesity or body mass index. Although body mass index is a poor measure of obesity, especially in the football player, it does provide some indicator of risk regarding heat illness. In several studies, linemen appear to be at a greater physiological strain than the smaller skill position players. Godek and colleagues (2008) reported that NFL linemen sweated at higher rates and lost larger volumes of sweat than skill position players, but did not lose greater weight due to significantly greater fluid intakes and less urine loss. In a study on NCAA Division I football players, increases in exercise intensity during practice were associated with greater elevations in core body temperature (DeMartini-Nolan et al., 2018). No differences were noted between linemen and skill position players in heart rate and body temperature. However, the amount of time spent at a higher intensity of exercise was significantly greater in the skill position players, suggesting that the heat strain for linemen was much greater and that the similar thermal strain was primarily related to the difference in exercise intensity between positions.

Strategies to Reduce Risk for Heat Illness

There have been a number of strategies discussed for reducing the risk for exertional heat illness. Conditioning, acclimatization, altering practice intensity and duration, and modifying uniform ensembles are all factors that have been considered in regard to reducing risk for heat illness. Another important consideration is cooling. The use of water baths following football practice is an effective and most efficient method of rapidly cooling core temperature (McDermott et al., 2009). To maximize the cooling effect, players need to remove their pads prior to entering the water (Miller et al., 2015).

The Effect of Cold Weather on Football Performance

In contrast to the number of studies conducted on American football players in the heat, the number of examinations on football in the cold is very limited. This is likely related to the relatively low number of cold-related injuries attributed to football players in cold weather conditions. Although it is not common, the risk of hypothermia does exist, and the risk of injury to exposed skin is still possible. It does require an appreciation for the potential risk, especially in games that are played in certain regions of the country. Many teams that play in such conditions generally have indoor practice facilities or indoor stadiums. However, there are several teams, whose tradition, or perhaps budget, maintain their games in outdoor venues. One example of a team that fits this mode is the Green Bay Packers. The coldest game played in NFL history is referred to as the *Ice Bowl*, the 1967 NFL championship game between the Dallas Cowboys and Green Bay Packers was played in Green Bay, Wisconsin. The game-time temperature was −13°F (−25°C) with a windchill of −36°F (−37.8°C).

Exposure to cold temperature results in a transfer of heat from the body to the environment. Heat loss occurs through either conductive or convective mechanisms. As ambient temperature drops below that of the body's core temperature, a gradient is developed that results in a loss of body heat. The difference between body temperature and the environment can be further magnified by wind speed. Wind can accelerate heat loss by removing warm air trapped in insulative clothing, increase evaporative cooling when insulative material is wet, and increase evaporative cooling directly from the skin when the skin is wet (Cheung, 2009). The term windchill is used to describe the combined effects of cold ambient temperature and air movement. Although a windchill index has been developed to reflect the relative risk of freezing-tissue injuries (see Hoffman, 2014 for further discussion), it is limited only to the risk of exposed skin freezing, not well-insulated skin. Most players competing in cold weather are able to insulate themselves with warm-weather gear and reduce that risk.

What Is the Physiological Effect of Playing in the Cold?

Playing football in the cold, whether it is cold, dry or cold, wet conditions, results in a physiological response that is focused on maintaining thermal homeostasis. Exposure to a cold environment results in a decrease in core body temperature due to the rapid transfer of heat from the core to the periphery. To defend core temperature, peripheral blood vessels constrict. Vasoconstriction appears to occur when skin temperature falls below 95°F (35°C) and becomes maximal when skin temperature drops below 88°F (31°C) (Veicteinas et al., 1982). Insulating the skin is an important countermeasure. In addition, an increase in metabolic heat production occurs through shivering. For the football player, the greatest increase in heat production occurs by playing the game itself. Muscular contraction occurring during the game will be the primary method of increasing thermogenesis (Toner and McArdle, 1988).

Although shivering is effective in increasing metabolic heat production, being active is the best way to maintain thermal homeostasis. For football players who are starting or will get regular playing time, the physical activity will be effective in maintaining core body temperature. In fact, playing the game of football itself during a cold stress likely generates enough metabolic heat so that shivering is not needed. It has been previously demonstrated that core temperature could be maintained within 0.9°F (0.5°C) when exercise is performed at ambient temperatures ranging between 32°F and 95°F (0°C and 35°C) (Claremont et al., 1975). When properly insulated, exercise in temperatures as low as −22°F (−30°C) may be sustained without significant changes in core temperature (Toner and McArdle, 1988). However, for players who are not playing, hypothermia (e.g., low body temperature) does become an issue if not protected.

In exposed skin, the vasoconstrictor response will help reduce heat loss and defend core temperature. However, this results in a decline in skin and muscle temperatures. Cold-induced vasoconstriction has pronounced effects on exposed skin, especially the hands and fingers, making them particularly susceptible to cold injury and a loss of manual dexterity (Brajkovic and Ducharme, 2003). This has important implications for the football player, especially skill position players. Interestingly, the larger players (i.e., linemen) may not suffer as much in the cold as the skill position players. The greater body fat common to linemen (see Chapter 4) may actually be beneficial during cold exposure. Individuals with a higher percentage of body fat appear to have a greater ability to maintain their core body temperature than their leaner individuals. A positive linear relationship has been demonstrated between body fat composition and core temperature during cold exposures (Toner et al., 1986). The high levels of subcutaneous fat have a greater insulatory ability, which limits the transfer of heat from the core of the body to the periphery by decreasing the rate of heat conduction.

Can a Football Player Acclimatize to Playing in the Cold?

This is an interesting question that doesn't have a definitive answer. The study of acclimatization to the cold has been relatively ignored compared to the extensive literature found on heat acclimatization. Part of the issue is that teams that play in cold environments generally have indoor practice facilities. The moment that practice is in a controlled temperate environment, the ability to adapt to a cold stress is removed. Playing once per week in the cold will not provide any ability for the body to adapt. However, for players who are chronically exposed to the cold, some degree of physiological adaptation may occur. An increase in tolerance to cold exposure may occur from two potential physiological adaptations. One adaptation is related to an increase in metabolic heat production through an exaggerated shivering response, while the other adaptation is thought to be related to an enhanced sympathetic response, resulting in a more rapid vasoconstriction of the skin (Sawka and Young, 2000). Interestingly, the enhanced sympathetic response has been suggested to be involved with a greater "toughness" that may be demonstrated in athletes tolerating cold environments (Dienstbier, 1991). In comparison to heat acclimatization, adaptation to chronic cold exposure develops at a much slower pace, reducing its effectiveness in preventing a cold injury (Hoffman, 2014).

Does Playing in the Cold Affect Football Performance?

As discussed in Chapter 1, football is a strength/power sport that relies predominantly on the anaerobic energy system. As such, the potential for a game to be negatively affected by being played in the cold weather exists. The ability to generate maximal strength and power is related to muscle temperature. When exercise is performed in a cold environment, muscle temperatures may decline. In laboratory-controlled experiments, decreases in muscle temperature ($-14°F$ [$-8°C$]) were demonstrated to reduce jump power by 43% (Davies and Young, 1983) and increase time to peak force (Davies et al., 1982; Davies and Young, 1983). The extent of power and force decrements is associated with the magnitude of muscle temperature reduction. Power outputs have been reported to decrease 3–6% for every 1.8°F (1°C) reduction in muscle temperature (Bergh and Ekblom, 1979; Sargeant, 1987). However, this may be related to the velocity of movement. Howard and colleagues (1994) reported that decrements in both peak torque and average power during cold exposure only occurred at contraction speeds greater than $180° s^{-1}$. At slower velocities of joint movement ($0° s^{-1}$ and $30° s^{-1}$), no significant differences were reported. To relate this to a football game, the cold weather may not effect offensive and defensive linemen to the same extent as skill position players because the linemen rarely reach high rates of speed due to a quick engagement with their opponent. However, acceleration or change in direction that is so important for skill position players may be affected. The mechanism that may contribute to these performance decrements in the skill position players may be related to a decrease in the rate of myofilament cross-bridge formation (Godt and Lindly, 1982;

Stein et al., 1982), reduction in nerve conduction velocity (Montgomery and MacDonald, 1990), and a possible change in motor unit recruitment patterns (Rome, 1990). As muscle temperatures decrease, the rate of muscle enzyme activity may also decrease, resulting in a reduced ability to replenish high-energy phosphates (Ferretti, 1992). Most of these mechanisms are speculative, especially in the football player. However, if the athlete is able to maintain muscle temperature by wearing appropriate cold-weather clothing, these decrements are likely avoided.

One of the major issues related to performance in cold-weather environments is the effect it has on manual dexterity. This is very relevant to skill position players such as wide receivers, running backs, and quarterbacks who need to be able catch and throw the football with precision. When skin temperatures fall to 20°C, an increase in pain sensation is felt, and when skin temperature declines to 15°C, a decrease in manual dexterity becomes apparent (Heus et al., 1995). As temperatures decrease, the cooling of superficial tissues in the fingers and hands are accompanied by decreases in joint mobility. As temperature drops further (below 7°C), tactile sensitivity becomes reduced (Kenefick et al., 2008). The duration of cold exposure experienced by uncovered skin is related to the magnitude of performance loss. Longer exposures result in greater declines in performance as muscles and nerves will continue to cool. Finger temperature has been demonstrated to be maintained by covering the face during cold-weather activity by wearing a balaclava (O'Brien et al., 2011). However, prolonged exposure with uncovered hands will still result in performance decrements.

What Are the Medical Concerns With Playing in the Cold?

Most injuries related to cold ambient temperatures are the result of prolonged exposure without proper clothing. Cold injuries among athletes engaged in competitive or recreational sports are rare. Players are generally able to maintain body temperature in the cold by wearing layers of clothing as insulation; wearing bulky insulative clothing though can hinder freedom of motion, critical for the football player. However, there have been many technological advances in clothing design to preserve core body temperature, while maintaining movement capabilities. If athletes decide to keep a certain part of their bodies exposed (e.g., offensive linemen exposing their arms), this can place them at an increased risk of cold injuries.

There are several injuries common to prolonged cold exposure. Hypothermia and frostbite are the most dangerous of the cold injuries. Immersion foot and chilblain are also common, but pose much less threat to survival. Hypothermia is defined as a lowering of the core body temperature below 95°F (35°C) (Ward et al., 1995). Core temperature of 90–95°F (32–35°C) is considered to be mild hypothermia, whereas core temperature below 90°F (32°C) is considered to be severe hypothermia. If exposure to a cold environment is of short duration, but the body is unable to maintain core temperature despite maximum heat production, the subsequent hypothermia is classified as acute hypothermia. When prolonged activity in the cold is accompanied by exhaustion and depletion of energy reserves, the ability to maintain core temperature is diminished and the ensuing hypothermia is classified as subacute (Ward et al., 1995). The primary difference between acute and subacute hypothermia is that during acute hypothermia, the body still has the capability of heat production, but the cold stress far exceeds the body's ability to maintain warmth. During subacute hypothermia, the body is able to maintain core temperature but is unable to maintain heat production because of prolonged activity and subsequent exhaustion to the body. To date, there has not been a single case report published of hypothermia in a football player. Likely, the duration of cold exposure and the ability of the player to wear appropriately insulated clothing minimize the risk for this serious injury.

Football players may be more susceptible to a freezing injury of exposed skin. As ambient temperature drops toward the freezing point, exposed skin becomes numb and loses its sense of touch and pain. This is accompanied by a transient general vasoconstriction. As ambient temperature continues to drop below freezing, the skin will actually freeze. Several injuries are associated with freezing of the skin. The extent of these injuries depends on the environmental temperature, wind velocity, and duration of exposure. If exposure results in only the superficial layers of the skin becoming frozen, *frostnip* is considered to have occurred. Frostnip is not associated with any subsequent damage or tissue loss and is not considered to be a serious cold injury. During frostnip, the skin may appear red and scaly. Sensation in the affected areas may be lost, but the skin still remains pliable. Once rewarmed, the affected areas may appear similar to first-degree sunburn. *Superficial frostbite* is the result of freezing of the skin and subcutaneous tissues. Although the skin is frozen, the deep underlying tissues remain pliable. Rewarming should be rapid in nature. After rewarming, the skin swells and becomes mottled blue or purple. If the deeper structures (muscle, bone, and tendons) of the exposed skin become frozen, the more serious *deep frostbite* is said to have occurred. The affected area is insensitive and becomes hard and fixed over joints (nonpliable). The color of the skin may be grayish purple or white marble, and actual crystallization of tissue fluids in the skin or subcutaneous tissues occurs. Although the tissue is frozen, movement in the affected body part may still occur because the tendons are not as sensitive to the cold as other tissue (Ward et al., 1995), and the primary muscle groups are at a distance from the area of injury. To date, there has been only one report of frostbite in a high school football player (Rivlin et al., 2014). However, that injury had little to do with environmental conditions. The player's finger was injured and the cold gel pack applied to the site of injury apparently contributed to the frostbite injury.

Both immersion foot and chilblain are related to prolonged exposure to cold and wet environments. There are no reports of this occurring in football players, and it is more often seen in individuals whose feet are immersed in water for several hours or days, such as a soldier. The cold-related injuries that may be common to sports such as mountaineering are not a threat to the football player. This is related to the athlete's ability to insulate himself sufficiently to maintain thermal homeostasis, and the duration of cold exposure is not long enough to cause significant cold injury. Even with exposed skin, the duration of cold exposure during a game or practice will always be short and the athlete's ability to rewarm exposed skin will reduce the risk. In addition, the metabolic heat generated during the game contributes to the maintenance of thermal homeostasis. Although cold injuries are not common to the football player, playing in the cold may make the football player more susceptible to common football injuries.

Lawrence and colleagues (2016) examined the effect of meteorological conditions on injury patterns in NFL players over two seasons. They compared four different temperature ranges: $\geq 21.0°C$ ($\geq 69.8°F$); $16.9-20.8°C$ ($62.4-69.4°F$); $10-16.7°C$ ($50-62.1°F$); and $\leq 9.7°C$ ($\leq 49.5°F$). Results indicated that the risk of concussion was significantly greater (twofold greater) during games played at a mean game-day temperature of $\leq 9.7°C$ ($\leq 49.5°F$) compared with a mean game-day temperature of $\geq 21.0°C$ ($\geq 69.8°F$). In addition, players were at a significantly greater risk for ankle injuries (1.5-fold greater) in games played at a mean game-day temperature of $\leq 9.7°C$ ($\leq 49.5°F$) compared with a mean game-day temperature of $\geq 21.0°C$ ($\geq 69.8°F$). No other significant effects were noted.

The Effect of Altitude on Football Performance

On October 2, 2005, the New Orleans Saints played the Philadelphia Eagles at Azteca Stadium in Mexico City. The game was played at 7,280 feet above sea level. The Saints play their home games at a stadium that is 3 feet above sea level, while the Eagles home field is 10 feet above sea level. Obviously, no team had a physiological advantage in regard to altitude exposure. However, was the player's performance at this altitude affected? More importantly, did playing at this altitude cause any health risk to the players? Most teams in the NFL or in college and high school sports play and practice at altitudes that are close to sea level. The New England Patriots play at 256 feet above sea level, while both the New York Jets and New York Giants practice and play their games at 7 feet above sea level. The Florida teams (Miami Dolphins, Tampa Bay Buccaneers, and the Jacksonville Jaguars) play at 4.3–36 feet above sea level. However, the Denver Broncos practice and play their home games at 5,280 feet above sea level. Could that be a true home field advantage?

As one ascends above sea level, the barometric pressure is reduced relative to the magnitude of the elevation. Because the weight of the upper atmosphere compresses the air of the lower atmosphere, barometric pressure decreases rapidly as one ascends from sea level. Changes in pressure also influence changes in ambient temperature. During ascent, the atmospheric pressure continuously decreases; however, the composition of the air remains the same as it was at sea level (20.93% oxygen, 0.03% carbon dioxide, and 79.04% nitrogen). The partial pressure of each gas is however reduced in direct proportion to the increase in altitude. The reduced partial pressure of oxygen (PO_2) results in a reduced pressure gradient, which impedes oxygen diffusion from the blood to the tissues. In addition to reduced oxygen availability as one ascends, there are other environmental issues that occur that can impact performance. Ambient temperature drops at a rate of 1.8°F (1°C) for every 490 feet (150 m) of ascent. So a game in Denver, Colorado, is also associated with a 19.4°F (10.8°C) drop in temperature. In addition to a reduction in ambient temperature during ascent to altitude, the amount of water vapor per unit volume of gas is also reduced. At high altitudes, even if the air was fully saturated with water, the actual amount of water vapor is very small. For example, at 68°F (20°C), the water vapor pressure is 17 mmHg, but at −4°F (−20°C), the corresponding water vapor pressure is only 1 mmHg. Thus, the extremely low humidity seen at altitude results in a large evaporative heat loss caused by ventilation of the dry inspired air. The risk of dehydration at altitude is great even at rest, but during exercise when the ventilation rate is further elevated, the risk becomes greater. Games played at altitude do require the athlete and training staff to be more cognizant of the need for hydrating frequently. Detailed discussion of hydration appears in Chapter 5.

What Is the Physiological Response to a Football Game Played at Altitude?

The primary physiological concern with playing a football game at altitude is the change in oxygen availability to the tissues. Reduction in oxygen levels, whether in arterial blood, inspired gases, or tissues, is known as *hypoxia*. Acute hypoxia, which occurs when an individual is initially exposed to altitude, results in changes in various physiological systems in the body. Most discussions on hypoxia cover altitudes up to and including 25,000 feet (7,600 m). Considering that the highest altitude that a game has been played is 7,280 feet, this section will focus on the physiological effects occurring at low to moderate altitudes. However, the reader should be aware of the severe physiological limitations seen at higher elevations. Figure 2.2 provides an overview of the physiological changes that may be experienced by football players as they ascend to a moderate altitude. The figure focuses on NFL teams, but the reader can apply this chart to any playing site to examine potential risks. It is important to understand that there is considerable variability in the response between athletes. Most changes observed at moderate altitudes involve the central nervous system. At 4,900 feet (1,500 m), night vision becomes impaired. At about 6,600 feet (2,000 m), resting heart rate becomes elevated and continues to elevate as ascent continues.

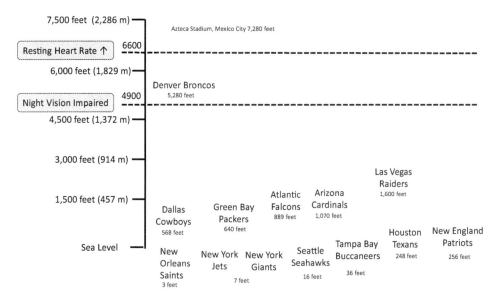

FIGURE 2.2 Physiological Changes at Low to Moderate Altitudes.

During ascents above sea level to approximately 9,800 feet (3,000 m), most individuals do not experience any noticeable symptoms while at rest.

As one ascends above sea level, the partial pressure of oxygen (PO_2) becomes reduced. To compensate for the reduced PO_2 at altitude, breathing rate is increased. The increase in ventilation does not appear to occur until inspired PO_2, which is approximately 160 mmHg at sea level, is reduced to approximately 100 mmHg. This is equivalent to an elevation of about 9,800 feet (3,000 m) (Ward et al., 1995). Although this is variable among individuals, for healthy competitive athletes such as football players, there is no physiological limitation in respiration as one plays at the highest altitudes (e.g., Denver or Mexico City). However, a concern as one plays at the higher altitudes such as Mexico City is the change in the pressure gradient between arterial PO_2 and tissue PO_2. At sea level, it is approximately 64 mmHg (the difference between an arterial PO_2 of 104 mmHg and a tissue PO_2 of 40 mmHg). This pressure gradient causes oxygen to rapidly diffuse into the tissues. However, a reduction in arterial PO_2 at altitude results in a decrease in the pressure gradient, which decreases the diffusion capability of oxygen from the vasculature into the tissue. At an altitude of 8,200 feet (2,500 m), the arterial PO_2 drops to about 60 mmHg, while the tissue PO_2 remains at 40 mmHg, thus creating a pressure gradient of only 20 mmHg. This 70% reduction in the pressure gradient causes a significant reduction in the speed at which oxygen moves between the capillaries and tissues.

Arriving and playing at altitude can result in an increase in cardiac output both at rest and during exercise. This is a compensation for the reduced oxygen availability caused by the lower PO_2. The primary mechanism resulting in the elevated cardiac output appears to be an increase in heart rate. Heart rate may increase 40–50% at rest without any change in stroke volume (Vogel and Harris, 1967). Even during exercise, the increase in cardiac output appears to be primarily the result of an increase in heart rate. In contrast to what is normally seen during exercise at sea level, stroke volume decreases during exercise at altitude (Vogel and Harris, 1967). This decrease is caused by a reduction in plasma volume that is observed within a short time after arrival at altitude (Singh et al., 1990). Initial exposure to altitude is also associated with diuresis and natriuresis (Honig, 1983). Diuresis may be explained by the evaporative heat loss caused by ventilation of dry inspired air at altitude, and natriuresis (increased sodium excretion in urine) appears to result from a decrease in the reabsorption of sodium in the kidneys due to the hypoxic stimulus (Honig, 1983).

What Are the Potential Effects of Altitude on Football Performance?

The 1968 Olympics was held in Mexico City [elevation 7,300 feet, (2,240 m)]. Numerous sprinting, jumping, and throwing records were set. These records were believed to be the benefit of a decrease in drag associated with the thinner air. Drag is the resistance that acts on a body in motion, either in air or in water. At altitude, the thinner air reduces the effects of drag, which results in faster times and a reduced energy cost. The performance benefits of a reduced drag for the football player may be expressed by an increase in the distance for field goals, punts, and passing.

Research examining the effect of altitude on anaerobic sports such as football does not appear to exist. Acute exposure to moderate altitude can result in a decrease in buffering capacity, and lower lactic acid concentrations seen during maximal exercise at altitude may be suggestive of potential performance decrements. However, there is no evidence to support this hypothesis. There is evidence, although in soccer, that performance at low to moderate altitudes (1,200–1703 m [4,000–5,750 feet]) will result in significant declines in the total distance covered during a game in elite soccer players (Nassis, 2013). A subsequent study by Bohner and colleagues (2015) confirmed these results by reporting significant reductions in total distance per minute and total distance of high intensity runs per minute in NCAA Division I soccer players competing at a moderate altitude (1,839 m [6033 feet]). Other studies examining sports, perhaps more similar to football in regard to physicality, reported significant performance decrements in repetitive explosive power and time for 20-m shuttle speed in senior club-level rugby players competing at 1,550 m (5,085 feet) (Hamlin et al., 2008). However, no change in choice reaction time was noted in rugby players competing at 1,600 m (5,249 feet) (O'Carroll and MacLeod, 1997). Evidence to date suggests that acute exposure to altitude may negatively affect the ability of athletes to perform repetitive high-intensity activity. However, this may be alleviated if athletes arrive at altitude several days prior to competition.

Can an Athlete Acclimatize to Competition at a Low to Moderate Altitude?

During prolonged altitude exposure, physiological adaptations that enhance the ability to perform at high elevations gradually occur. However, these adaptations never reach the point that fully compensates for hypobaric hypoxia. Although several physiological systems in the body are able to adapt to altitude, these systems have different time courses for adaptation, and can be reviewed at much greater depth elsewhere (Hoffman, 2014). However, in contrast to a sojourn to Mount Everest, the football player does not have an extended period of time to acclimatize to a game being played at a low to moderate elevation. Certain adaptations do occur fairly quickly. Short-term exposure (24 h) to altitude (between 1,780 m [5,840 feet] and 2,800 m [9,186 feet]) has been shown to result in a relatively quick increase in erythropoietin production that can be sustained for 6 h postexposure (Ge et al., 2002). However, most physiological adaptations to short-term altitude acclimatization programs appear to benefit endurance performance. For acclimatization to occur, training should occur between 4,900 and 9,800 feet (1,500 and 3,000 m), with the lower range thought to be the lowest elevation at which an acclimatization effect will occur (Hoffman, 2014). It is recommended that athletes arrive at least two weeks prior to competition and ideally four to six weeks prior to competition. This is not realistic for any football team. In addition, there is no evidence to show that acclimatization will benefit a football team.

Is There a Performance Disadvantage by Playing at Altitude?

College and professional football teams may have to play a game or two per year at a location that may be considered to be at a low to moderate altitude. Does playing there pose a distinct disadvantage? It is an interesting question, because the home team has had the time to acclimatize to the altitude, and the visiting team arrives perhaps 24–48 h prior to the game. One way to potentially examine whether a home field advantage is to compare the Denver Broncos to

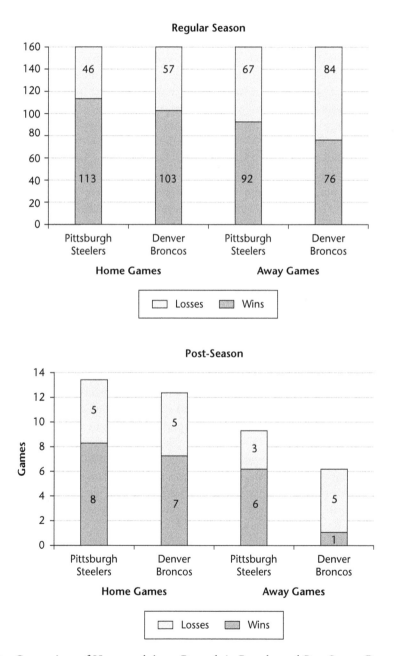

FIGURE 2.3   Comparison of Home and Away Records in Regular and Post-Season Between Pittsburgh Steelers and Denver Broncos.

another team that has been successful over time. The Denver Broncos are the only team in the NFL that plays at a low to moderate altitude (5,280 feet [1,609 m]). As discussed earlier, this altitude does result in some minor physiological changes, but it has not been studied extensively. In the past 20 years, the Denver Broncos have an overall regular season record of 179–141 (a 55.9% winning percentage). However, closer examination of their home and away splits shows that they win at home 64.4% of the time (103–57), but on the road they are 76–84 (47.5%). On first glance, you can say that they have a large home field advantage. In fact, over the past 20 seasons, they have won more games at home than on the road in 14 of the 20 seasons. However, the NFL indicates that the home team wins between 55% and 60% of the time. So, does that 64.4% home winning percentage an advantage? Over 20 years playing their home games in Denver, Colorado, may have resulted in possibly 7–15 more home wins than the average NFL team. That is less than one win per year. Playoffs though tell a more interesting story. In the playoffs, the Broncos are 6–3 at home, but 0–4 on the road, and 1–1 at a neutral site (Super Bowl). The combination of a moderate altitude and freezing temperatures may be too much for teams that come from temperate climates at sea level. To provide further insight into whether playing in Denver provides any advantage, Figure 2.3 compares the home and away splits between the Broncos and the Pittsburgh Steelers for the past 20 years. The Steelers are one of the most storied franchises in the history of the NFL and won two Super Bowls during this time frame. As can be seen in the figure, the Steelers actually have a greater winning percentage at home than the Broncos, but they also have a winning percentage on the road. Considering that Denver loses more than they win away, perhaps they do have a stronger home field advantage compared to the rest of the league.

Are There Any Medical Concerns With Games Played at a Low to Moderate Altitude?

Altitude sickness is not an issue at low to moderate altitudes. However, there have been several studies focusing on whether games at a low to moderate altitude increase the risk for injury. Most of these studies have focused on the risk for concussion. The first study examined high school football players performing at altitudes ranging from 7 to 6,903 feet (median, 600 feet) (Smith et al., 2013). The study monitored concussion data for seven years. Results of the study indicated a 31.6% reduction in the incidence rate of concussions at an altitude above 645 feet. The mechanism suggested was related to a greater red blood cell mass from the chronic altitude exposure leading to greater intracranial volume and decreased compliance. Subsequent research published shortly thereafter on NFL players also reported a lower rate of concussion (30% lower risk) in NFL players competing 644 feet (196.3 m) above sea level (Myer et al., 2014). Those investigators speculated that physiological adaptation to higher altitude resulted in an increase in cerebral blood flow causing an increase in intracranial pressure providing greater protection. However, the biggest issue with this hypothesis is that there is only one location that is at an altitude that can stimulate adaptation (i.e., Denver, Colorado). Most other stadiums are at altitudes that afford little to any stimulus to altitude (Ge et al., 2002).

Even without a clear mechanism to support the lowered risk of concussion at higher altitudes of play, this was still a hot topic of research. In 2016, Lynall and colleagues (2016) examined the effect of altitude on concussion risk in NCAA college football players. They examined 21 NCAA Division I football programs for up to five years. A total of 169 concussions were recorded in 47 states. The sample median elevation for competitions was 178 m (range: 1–2,202 m). The concussion rate was greatest at the higher elevations. Using a median split, the concussion rate above 178 m was 1.47 times greater ($p = 0.01$) than below 178 m. In addition, concussion sustained at higher altitudes appeared to require a longer time for return to recovery compared to

TABLE 2.3 Effect of Different Altitudes on Concussion Rates in NFL Players

Home Field/Practice	Game Played	Exposures	Concussion Incidents	Rate (Concussion/ Exposures)
Low altitude ≤644 feet	Home (low altitude) ≤644 feet	1,180	363	0.31
	Away (high altitude) ≥644 feet	206	66	0.32
High altitude ≥644 feet	Home (high altitude) ≥644 feet	328	65	0.20*
	Away (low altitude) ≤644 feet	206	75	0.36

Source: Data from Connolly et al., 2018.

Note: * = significantly different (p < 0.05) from low–low and high–low groups.

concussions sustained at lower altitudes. However, little to no discussion was noted at concussion incidents at altitudes that physiological challenges would be apparent. It is difficult to state that an altitude of 178 m (584 feet) will result in a hypoxic challenge. Examples of teams that play at that altitude include Dallas Cowboys, Green Bay Packers, Atlanta Falcons, and Arizona Cardinals (see Figure 2.3). Games played at those venues cannot be considered to be played at altitude. Regardless, the results of this study called into question the previous results of both Smith et al. (2013) and Myer et al. (2014). A subsequent study analyzing concussions incidents in the NFL between the 2012 and 2015 seasons divided each incident into four quadrants (Connolly et al., 2018). A total of 1,920 team exposures were analyzed: 534 were observed at nine stadiums above 644 feet, while the remaining 1,386 exposures played below 644 feet. Four quartiles of elevation were examined: 0–19 feet, 20–397 feet, 398–704 feet, and 705–5280 feet. No differences were noted in concussion rate between any of these quartiles. When using the previous cutoff altitude of 644 feet (Myer et al., 2014), the investigators examined the effect of these teams playing home versus away (see Table 2.3). A team whose home field was above 644 feet and played at that elevation or higher was labeled high–high and their away games were labeled high–low. A team whose home field was below 644 feet and played their home games at that altitude or lower was labeled low–low and when they played at altitude they were labeled low–high. High–high was reported to have a lower rate of concussion than both low–high and high–low. In addition, a 28% reduction in concussion rate was reported for the high–high teams compared with the overall concussion incidence rate.

It appears that the initial studies suggesting that altitude may provide some degree of protection has not been supported in latter studies. The issue is more likely in the methodology and interpretation of what altitude is. There is only one stadium in the NFL that poses a physiological challenge, and that is in Denver. The other stadiums are at altitude that do not provide any hypoxic challenge, nor would they stimulate any altitude adaptation. Further highlighting this is the evidence presented by Lawrence and colleagues (2016) that reported no effect of altitude exposure on increasing the concussion incidence in NFL players. Further, altitude did not increase risk for ankle, knee, shoulder, or hamstring injuries as well.

What Is the Effect of Jet Lag on Football Performance?

Jet lag can be defined as a syndrome involving insomnia or excessive daytime sleepiness following travel across at least two time zones (American Academy of Sleep Medicine, 2005). In a study examining the effect of rapidly crossing multiple (six) time zones in an easterly direction, Wright and colleagues (1983) reported significant reductions in both strength and endurance. In addition, subjective feelings of fatigue, weakness, insomnia, headache, and irritability were reported. It took approximately five days for performance and subjective measures to return to baseline. Although most football teams do not cross six-time zones, the popularity of football internationally has now created annual games in Europe that do force athletes to cross multiple time zones. In a study examining the effect of time zone changes in NFL games, there was interest in determining whether there was a home field advantage in games that required extensive travel (Jehue et al., 1993). Travel by west coast teams to play east coast or centrally located teams generally cross two to three time zones. This means that a 1 p.m. game would start chronobiologically for these athletes at 10 or 11 a.m. West coast teams experienced a 19.7% change in winning percentage between home and away. The investigators indicated that the opposite direction of travel, east coast teams flying west, was not as detrimental and suggested that westward flights were more adaptable than easterly travel.

This question was revisited more than 20 years later by Roy and Forest (2018). They examined travel from coast to coast, in professional athletes, including NFL players. They reported a significant correlation between time zones crossed and winning percentage ($r = 0.34$, $p = 0.024$). In addition, analysis performed on the games played during the afternoon revealed no significant circadian advantage or disadvantage regardless of the direction of travel in the NFL. However, the winning percentage for NFL teams traveling westward and crossing three time zones was 22% for games played at night. These results indicate an advantage for teams playing closer to their circadian peak, highlighting the importance of circadian rhythms in sport performance.

The potential disadvantage of crossing three time zones, especially in a westward direction, may not just be a case of chronobiology, but of significant physiological alterations. Kraemer and colleagues (2016) examined the effect of a three time zone change (travel from Hartford, Connecticut to Los Angeles, California, and back) on performance and biochemical responses. They also examined the effect of a compression garment on providing a potential countermeasure to minimize the effect of the transmeridian flight. Participants performed testing prior to their travel to the west coast. They arrived performed additional testing and prepared for a simulated athletic contest the next day (day 2). Participants flew through the night back to Hartford landing on day 3 and performed additional assessments through day 5. Significant decreases were observed in power (countermovement jump) for all five days of the study. In addition, significant slower times for speed (40-yard sprint) and agility (pro-agility test) for four-days posttravel were noted. Speed and agility times returned to baseline levels by day 5. No differences were noted in hand grip strength. Participants who wore the compression garment experienced no significant declines in performance. Perceptions of fatigue were significantly elevated in the afternoon of the day they arrived in California and lasted until the morning of day 3, but returned by the afternoon of day 4. There were no differences observed between the groups. In addition, sleep disturbances were also noted on day 4 following the return flight back to Hartford, and no differences were noted between the groups.

The investigators also assessed the hormonal response to transmeridian travel (Kraemer et al., 2016). The investigators reported that higher melatonin values noted before the westbound trip were associated with better sleep quality perception by the participants, and the attenuated response observed at 0900 following the eastbound late night "overnight" flight and transport to the laboratory was associated with a much lower sleep quality from the prior night. Cortisol and testosterone concentrations were reported to be significantly elevated in both groups after the simulated sport competition. Testosterone was still elevated following the eastbound flight in both groups, suggesting a continued anabolic signaling response being maintained during the recovery period. The investigators did acknowledge that this peak may have been augmented by the typical diurnal response of testosterone, but that was not seen with cortisol.

In another publication from that study, Kupchak and colleagues (2017) investigated the effect of transmeridian travel on coagulation and fibrinolytic systems. Long flights increase the risk of developing venous thromboembolism due to extensive sitting, reduced oxygen flow, and low humidity. Sitting for an extended time is associated with a reduced velocity of venous blood flow in lower extremities and an increase in blood viscosity. Decreases in air pressure and the reduced oxygen flow in the airline's cabin can limit fibrinolytic activity and lead to venous stasis (Maher et al., 1976). The investigators reported significant elevations in both coagulation and fibrinolytic systems postexercise, and activation of coagulation continued following the transcontinental flight. Interestingly, the transcontinental flight alone did not activate the coagulation and fibrinolytic systems, but the acute exercise protocol was able to elicit a response on the blood hemostatic system, exhibited by the activation of the coagulation system. To provide balance to the hypercoagulable state, the fibrinolytic system was also reported to be activated. The wearing of a full-body compression garment did have a positive effect on coagulation and reduced the risk for potential clot formation on transcontinental travel.

Summary

This chapter demonstrated the effect of various environmental extremes on the health and performance of football players. The most common stressor to most football programs is the thermal strain common to summer conditioning and the early part of the football season. This is potentially the most dangerous part of the year for players and coaches need to be aware and make any necessary adjustments in practices to minimize risk of heat illness. Issues related to hypothermia need to be recognized, and players should be encouraged to wear insulated clothing and avoid exposing any skin in freezing temperatures. Altitude exposure is not common in football, but the potential for significant physiological changes does exist if games are played in a unique area. Evidence to date is not convincing that playing at altitude less than 6,000 feet provides any significant advantage or risk. However, further research is warranted in football. This is especially relevant with the greater number of international games being played. The greater number of international competitions also increases the importance of recognizing potential risks associated with traveling multiple time zones, and potential countermeasures that can be used to assist in recovery.

3

STRENGTH AND CONDITIONING FOR FOOTBALL

In 2012, a multiorganizational taskforce was charged with examining the rash of needless deaths emanating out of National Collegiate Athletic Association (NCAA) Division I football programs that had resulted in the death of 21 players in the previous ten years from either exertional heatstroke or sickle cell trait. The report "The Inter-Association Task Force for Preventing Sudden Death in Collegiate Conditioning Sessions: Best Practices Recommendations" was published later that year in the *Journal of Athletic Training* (Casa et al., 2012). The consensus of the broad array of medical, athletic training, and sport performance organizations such as the National Strength and Conditioning Association (NSCA) and the College Strength Coaches Conditioning Association (CSCCA) was the understanding that developing appropriately designed training programs can maximize sport performance for football players. It was emphasized that an effective strength and conditioning program relies on scientific principles of exercise science intended to stimulate improvements specific to the sport. This should be the basis of the conditioning program. The training culture in the ten years prior to the 2012 report indicated that athlete's development, health, and safety were overshadowed by a desire to enhance athlete toughness, discipline, and focus on success at all costs. Unfortunately, this environment created by a number of coaching staffs around the United States caused numerous but 100% preventable deaths in college football. The issues leading to these deaths were often the result of strength and conditioning coaches using conditioning as a punishment for a bad season, and coaches attempting to build mental toughness through inappropriate training sessions. Furthermore, it was believed that a poor understanding of program progression and setting unrealistic training goals by strength and conditioning coaches contributed to these needless deaths. In general, these coaches lacked the basic understanding of exercise science and the principles of training!

This chapter will provide an overview of the basic principles of training. It provides a review of exercise program development and focuses on the knowledge base that has been developed in the strength and conditioning of football players. Specific discussion will focus on off-season training, inseason training, various modalities of training (e.g., use of Olympic movements, Ballistic training), and training periodization. In addition, discussion will also focus on performance improvements during an athlete's career, with primary emphasis being on both high school and collegiate athletes. What this chapter will not do is provide a "recommended" training program for football. There are so many potential combinations of exercises and training paradigms that make it very difficult to state that one program is more appropriate than another. There are so many variables that can impact training program success; thus, it becomes imperative that the coach provides a scientific justification for the specific exercise prescription. If that occurs, the likelihood of success will be vastly improved and the risk for catastrophic injury will be significantly reduced.

Basic Principles of Training

It is expected that strength and conditioning coaches follow the basic principles of training. That is, program development adheres to the principles of specificity, overload, progression, individuality, diminishing returns, and reversibility (Hoffman, 2014). Figure 3.1 provides an overview of the basic principles of training. The *specificity principle* refers to the development of a training program that focuses on the specific physiological, biomechanical, and medical needs of the sport. It is the goal for all coaches that physical performance improvements directly relate to better football performance. However, the "carryover" effect from the weight room to the field is not 100%. Thus, a 10% improvement in strength or power does not equate to a 10% improvement in football playing ability. To maximize the carryover effect, it is critical that the exercises used and the energy system stressed are consistent with the movement patterns and energy system of the game. Thus, running 5 miles is going to focus on the aerobic energy system, it will have little impact on football playing performance.

The *overload principle* is focused on making the athlete train at a level that they are normally not accustomed to working at. The overload is what will stimulate physiological adaptation. However, this is where many mistakes in the exercise prescription occur. The object of this principle is to make appropriate adjustments to the training program that will provide a stress that is above what the athlete is used to. It is not to force the athlete to exercise at an intensity or a volume that risks their health and well-being. As the athlete adapts, adjustments are made accordingly and this is the basis of the *progression principle*: that the overload will progress as the athlete adapts. However, it is imperative that the coach understands that athletes progress at different rates leading to the important understanding of the *individuality principle*. Two athletes

Principles of Training

Principle of Training	Definition
Specificity	Adaptations are specific to the muscles trained, the intensity of the exercise performed, the metabolic demands of the exercise and the joint angle trained. Except for actual practice of sport – no conditioning program has 100% carryover. To maximize carryover exercises should be selected that simulate sport movement.
Overload	For training adaptations to occur, the muscle or physiological component being trained must be exercised at a level that it is not normally accustomed to.
Progression	Physiological adaptations results in performance improvements. As such, the relative intensity will change requiring that the exercise prescription be modified. This is more appropriately termed progressive overload.
Individuality	Refers to concept that athletes respond differently to the same training stimulus. Variability of the training response is likely related to genetic predisposition and pre-training status.
Principle of Diminishing Returns	Performance gains are related to the level of training experience of the athlete. Freshmen football players will likely experience greater gains in strength than senior football players.
Principle of Reversibility	When training stimulus is removed or reduced (e.g., that may occur due to injury), the ability of the athlete to maintain performance may become reduced, and eventually the effect of this detraining period will cause the prior performance gains to revert back to their original level.

FIGURE 3.1   Principles of Training.

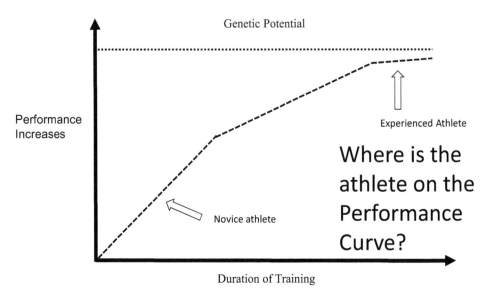

FIGURE 3.2 Performance Training Curve.

Source: Adapted from Hoffman, 2014.

performing the same training program will likely respond differently. That is the primary reason why coaches need to monitor their players on an individual basis and make changes according to the individual results observed. Figure 3.2 highlights the differences in rate of improvement of athletes with varying years of experience. Differences in performance improvements may not be related to a poor effort, laziness, or lack of toughness, but simply a different physiological capability related to genetics or training experience. Coaches need to recognize this and understand that pushing an athlete past their physiological limits may not only increase the risk for overtraining but may increase the risk of a catastrophic outcome related to exertional rhabdomyolysis, heatstroke, or a cardiovascular event. This may be exacerbated with an athlete that has sickle-cell trait (Anderson, 2017).

In the training facility, both young (e.g., first year players) and more experienced athletes will train together. The young players generally have less resistance training experience than the older players, who may be in their fourth or fifth year of competition. These younger players generally have a "greater window of adaptation" that will likely result in a greater response to the training program. This does not necessarily mean that the younger players worked harder than the older players, it is simply the reflection of training experience. That is the basis of the *principle of diminishing returns*. Simply, as you gain strength, power, or speed, your ability to generate further improvement is reduced. However, if you do not provide the appropriate training stimulus, the results can return to baseline level and this is what is referred to as the *principle of reversibility*. This can often be seen following injury, in which the athlete is unable to exercise for an extended period of time, which prevents/limits the athlete from maintaining the required training stimulus.

Exercise Program Development

The most difficult aspect in the development of the strength and conditioning program is the implementation of the entire program. The appropriate implementation of resistance training, sprint, and agility training and conditioning is crucial for maximizing performance gains at the appropriate time of the yearly program, while minimizing the risk for overtraining. This is obviously the major focus of periodization, whose theory and efficacy are covered in depth elsewhere (Issurin, 2016; Mujika et al., 2018; Williams et al., 2017), but it will be discussed in relation to football later in this chapter.

It is important to note that no single method of program prescription has universal acceptance. For a training program to be effective, it needs to be based on sound scientific evidence (Hoffman, 2014). The various training methods that exist simply give the strength and conditioning professional tools that can be used at the appropriate time in the yearly training cycle. Although there is often overlap, training programs are specific for each sport; thus, the examples in this chapter will be focused on American football.

Prior to any workout, the strength and conditioning professional must lead or direct a structured warm-up routine to prepare athletes for the subsequent workout. Proper warm-up routines can also reduce the risk for injury during training sessions. Although the use of static stretching exercises was the predominant method of the warm-up in previous generations, a dynamic warm-up that utilizes exercise-specific movement patterns has become more favorable and likely provides the greatest benefit in preparing the athlete for the training session (Opplert and Babault, 2018). It is important to note that the warm-up should not fatigue the athlete for subsequent performance. As athletes move from one training phase to another, it is imperative that they are physically ready for each proceeding phase. The acute program variables of intensity, volume, and exercise selection should progress to provide the necessary overload that can stimulate further adaptation in each subsequent training phase. Emphasis on proper technique should always be a priority. Load should not be emphasized until the athlete has demonstrated successful technique for the exercise.

In the development of the off-season training program for football, the strength and conditioning professional needs to set the training goals for the team and the individual athlete. Training goals for the team are often generic, regarding emphasis on hypertrophy (e.g., muscle growth), strength, or power. However, to optimize the training stimulus and maximize performance benefits, the coach will also need to focus on the individual athlete's strengths and weaknesses. This will allow the training program to be tailored for the specific athlete. Thus, the goals of the off-season training program can and should be general for the team and specific for each athlete. For example, the use of ballistic exercises (i.e., squat jump or bench press throws) may be more effective to install for an experienced football player than for the freshman player (Hoffman et al., 2005b). Coaches need to determine which training component has the greatest chance to stimulate further adaptation.

In general, the off-season training program for football progresses from developing muscle hypertrophy to focusing on strength, power, and speed. However, athletes also need to maintain a minimal level of conditioning. For many sports, this can be accomplished by playing their sport, this though is not possible for football players. These athletes may need to participate in activities such as playing pick-up basketball and racquet sports. The basis of all off-season training programs is to enhance the performance capability of the athlete primarily through increasing strength, power, and speed. In addition, a primary training goal for some football players may include altering body composition by increasing lean muscle mass and decreasing fat mass. At the beginning of the off-season training program, the football player will primarily be in the weight room. The resistance training program generally begins with a preparatory or hypertrophy phase of training that consists of high-volume (greater number of repetitions performed per set) and low-intensity (loads with a lower percentage of the athlete's 1-repetition maximum [1RM]) training. The purpose for this program is to prepare the players for the higher intensity lifting that will be performed during subsequent stages of the training program. The duration for this training phase is approximately four to five weeks. If the athlete is focused on increasing muscle size (may be common among younger athletes), this phase of training can be of longer duration. If the athlete's primary goal is to increase strength and power, then this phase will be used to prepare for more complicated exercises of higher intensity that will be incorporated into the later phases of the training program (Hoffman, 2014).

The next training phase during the off-season training program for football generally focuses on strength development. The intensity during this training phase increases as compared to the preparatory/hypertrophy phase, resulting in fewer repetitions performed per set. As a result, the total volume of training is decreased. During this training phase, additional exercises (primarily multiple-joint, structural movement exercises) can be incorporated into the training program to increase the training stimulus. The coach often incorporates Olympic-style lifting movements (e.g., high pulls) during this phase. These exercises could also appear during the initial phase of training, but inexperienced or novice athletes may benefit from developing a strength base and focusing on proper technique with the traditional power lifting exercises. In addition, the incorporation of these exercises in the latter phases of training provides a degree of variation to the training program that prevents monotony. This training phase is often four to six weeks in duration. During this training phase, plyometric exercises and/or speed and agility drills can also be integrated into the training program.

The next phase of training emphasizes more power production. During this training phase, intensity of exercise is elevated further and training volume is reduced further (keep in mind that there is an inverse relationship between training intensity and training volume – as intensity elevates, volume is reduced). For the collegiate football player, this phase may be interrupted by spring football. If this is the case, the athlete may enter a strength/maintenance program for the duration of spring football. If so, training intensity and training volume are generally reduced. Reductions in training volume can be accomplished by reducing the number of assistance exercises and/or number of sets. However, if an adjustment to the strength and conditioning program is not done, the added load of the spring practice schedule may increase the risk for overtraining. Following spring football, the strength and conditioning professional can begin the resistance training program again from the hypertrophy or preparatory phase before proceeding to the other training phases. This may assist the athlete in recovering from spring football.

During the strength/power phase, a greater emphasis is placed on Olympic and ballistic exercises, especially for the experienced, resistance-trained football player. Exercises, such as the snatch, power clean, and push press, are often added to the program, while some of the traditional power lifting exercises or assistance exercises are removed. Previous research has shown that Olympic exercises can enhance speed and power development in resistance-trained athletes during their off-season training program to a greater extent than the traditional power lifting exercises (Hoffman et al., 2004a). This will be discussed in greater detail later in the chapter. In addition, a speed and agility program is often included during this training phase. These exercises generally do not result in a change to the resistance training program and are compatible for this training phase.

During the power phase of training, a speed and agility routine is often incorporated into the weekly routine of the football player. It is important to recognize that speed and agility training is not intended to enhance the athlete's conditioning. Although it does help and if properly designed, it can contribute to improving the fitness level of the football player, the work-to-rest interval is relatively longer than one would expect when goals include conditioning. For example, the work-to-rest ratio for an exercise that enhances anaerobic capacity may be 1:4; however, when focusing on the quality per repetition, the work-to-rest ratio can elongate to 1:8 (Hoffman, 2014). The focus of agility, speed, and plyometric exercises is on the quality of work, and

TABLE 3.1 Off-Season Resistance Training Program (Four-Days per Week, Split Routine)

Preparatory/Hypertrophy Phase (4–6 Weeks)		Strength Phase (4–6 Weeks)		Strength/Power Phase (4–6 Weeks)		Peaking Phase (4 Weeks)	
★ = core exercises 1.4 × 8–10 repetitions per set		★ = core exercises 1.4 × 6–8 repetitions per set		★ = core exercises 1.4 × 4–6 repetitions per set		★ = core exercises 1.5 × 1–3 repetitions per set	
Assistance exercise 3 × 8–10 repetitions per set		Assistance exercise 3 × 6–8 repetitions per set		Assistance exercise 3 × 4–6 repetitions per set		Rest between sets: 3 min	
Rest between sets: 1 min		Rest between sets: 3 min		Rest between sets: 3 min			
Days 1 + 3	*Days 2 + 4*	*Days 1 + 3*	*Days 2 + 4*	*Days 1 + 3*	*Days 2 + 4*	*Days 1 + 3*	*Days 2 + 4*
Squat*	Bench press*	Squat*	High pulls*	Squat*	High pulls/power clean*	Power cleans (floor)/snatch (floor)*	Hang cleans/hang snatches (waist)
Leg extension	Inclined bench press	Dead lifts	Bench press*	Dead lifts/snatch*	Bench press*	Squat*	Bench press*
Leg curl	Dumbbell incline fly	Leg curls	Inclined bench press	Leg curl	Inclined bench press	Box jumps*	Push jerk/push press*
Standing calf raise	Seated shoulder press*	Standing calf raise	Dumbbell incline fly	Lateral pulldown*	Push press/push jerk*	Seated row*	Power shrugs*
Lateral pulldown*	Upright row	Lateral pulldown*	Seated shoulder press*	Seated row*	Front/lateral raise	Dumbbell biceps curl (3 × 4–6)	Triceps pushdown (3 × 4–6)
Seated row*	Front/lateral raise	Seated row*	Front/lateral raise	Dumbbell biceps curl (3 × 4–6)	Triceps pushdown	Abdominal routine (3 × 20)	Abdominal routine (3 × 20)
Dumbbell biceps curl	Triceps pushdown	Dumbbell biceps curl	Triceps pushdown	Barbell biceps curl	Abdominal routine (3 × 20)		
Barbell biceps curl	Triceps extension	Barbell biceps curl	Triceps extension	Hyperextension			
Hyperextension	Sit-ups (3 × 20)	Hyperextension	Sit-ups (3 × 20)	Abdominal routine (3 × 20)			
Crunch (3 × 20)		Crunch (3 × 20)					

Seventy-two hours between days 1 and 3 and between days 2 and 4. Days 1 and 2 and days 3 and 4 can be performed consecutively. For instance, this split-routine training program can be performed on Monday, Tuesday, Thursday, and Friday (four days per week).

not on the quantity. As the athlete moves into the later stages of the off-season training program, the speed and agility work become more *up-tempo* to contribute to aspects of anaerobic conditioning. However, a longer work-to-rest ratio still requires 100% effort for each drill.

The final phase of the off-season training program for football is the peaking phase. During this training phase, the exercise intensity is at its highest, while training volume is reduced further. During this training phase, the football player focuses on getting into peak condition for the start of preseason training camp. The lower training volume provides the player with additional time to focus on anaerobic conditioning exercises. During the final two to three weeks of the strength/power phase and throughout the peaking phase, the football player's focus will be on getting into peak anaerobic condition to play a competitive football season.

Table 3.1 provides an example of an off-season resistance training program for a football team, while Table 3.2 depicts an eight-week anaerobic conditioning program for preparing football players for the competitive season. This program is an example whose efficacy can be supported by scientific evidence. However, there are a multitude of combinations having

TABLE 3.2 Off-Season Anaerobic Conditioning Program

	Monday	Tuesday	Wednesday	Thursday	Friday	Saturday
Week 1		Agility and form running	2 × 200 m, 5 × 60 m sprints	Agility and form running	1 × line drill, 2 × intervals	
Week 2		Agility and form running	4 × 200 m, 6 × 60 m sprints	Agility and form running	1 × line drill, 3 × intervals	
Week 3	4 × starts 3 × intervals	Agility and form running	4 × 200 m, 6 × 60 m sprints	Agility and form running	1 × line drill, 3 × intervals	4 × 200 m, 4 × 100 m, 4 × 40 m sprints
Week 4	6 × starts 3 × intervals	Agility and form running	5 × 200 m, 8 × 60 m sprints	Agility and form running	2 × line drill, 3 × intervals	4 × 200 m, 4 × 100 m, 4 × 40 m sprints
Week 5	8 × starts 4 × intervals	Agility and form running	6 × 200 m, 8 × 60 m sprints	Agility and form running	2 × line drill, 4 × intervals	5 × 200 m, 5 × 100 m, 5 × 40 m sprints
Week 6	10 × starts 4 × intervals	Agility and form running	7 × 200 m, 10 × 60 m sprints	Agility and form running	3 × line drill, 4 × intervals	5 × 200 m, 5 × 100 m, 5 × 40 m sprints
Week 7	10 × starts 5 × intervals	Agility and form running	8 × 200 m, 10 × 60 m sprints	Agility and form running	3 × line drill, 4 × intervals	6 × 200 m, 6 × 100 m, 6 × 40 m sprints
Week 8	10 × starts 6 × intervals	3 × line drill	8 × 200 m, 10 × 60 m sprints	Agility and form running	Rest	Report to camp

Notes: Starts – 10-m sprint from 3-point football stance; intervals – run on an oval track, sprint the straightaways (100 m), and jog the turns (100 m); line drill – a shuttle run of goal line to 10-yard line and back, goal line to 20-yard line and back, goal line to 30-yard line and back, and finally goal line to 40-yard line and back; agility and form running include specific drills to enhance change of direction and speed. Form running is focused more on sprint running technique.

similar or greater efficacy that can be used. This program should be examined in the context that there is no spring football. It was a program that was developed and used for a NCAA Division III institution, which did not permit physical contact period during spring football. As a result, the team was trained through the limited spring football period. An argument could be made that this is the best way of preparing football players for the upcoming season. It is difficult at times to understand the importance of putting the pads on during the spring and risk losing key players to injury, when they have yet reached peak condition. Previous research has shown that a large proportion of injuries that occur in spring practices are the result of full-contact drills (Steiner et al., 2016). The emphasis on getting ready for spring football may have been a potential reason for some of the inappropriate training programs used during the onset of the off-season conditioning program that resulted in several catastrophic outcomes. During the same period of time in which more than 20 NCAA Division I athletes have died, only one NFL player has died due to heatstroke (Korey Stringer of the Minnesota Vikings in 2001 at the age of 27) during summer training camp. Most interesting is that the NFL has limited contact time in the off-season, and it doesn't appear to diminish their ability to prepare their players for a grueling 16-game schedule. There does not seem to be any compelling or justifiable reason for full-contact spring football. However, meetings, teaching sessions, and limited drills should be employed, but not at the expense of the off-season strength and conditioning program.

Efficacy of Off-Season Strength and Conditioning Programs for Football

There have been a number of studies that have examined the relationship between strength, speed, and power on football playing performance (Hoffman, 2008). Discussion of these investigations appears in Chapter 4. The magnitude of performance improvements during both inseason and off-season training has been studied less frequently. Most studies that have focused on this question generally compare different acute program variables such as training frequency, modes of exercise, and/or types of training programs using different periodization paradigms. These studies will be the focus of this section.

One of the initial studies examining performance changes during off-season conditioning programs in football analyzed the effect of training frequency (Hoffman et al., 1990). The study was conducted at the University of Connecticut and compared the effect of a three-day, four-day, five-day, and six-day resistance training program on body mass, strength, speed, and vertical jump height during a ten-week off-season training program. Sixty-one players self-selected their training frequency. The players in the three-day per week group performed no more than three exercises per body part, and performed all body parts per workout. The players in the four-day per week group performed a two-day split routine, in which at least three exercises for the chest, shoulders, and triceps were performed on Mondays and Thursdays and exercises for the legs, back, and biceps were performed on Tuesdays and Fridays. Players in the five-day per week group performed three exercises for chest, legs, and triceps three days per week (Mondays, Wednesdays, and Fridays), while performing shoulders, back, and biceps on Tuesdays and Thursdays. Players in the six-day per week group performed four exercises for the chest, legs, shoulders, and triceps on Mondays, Tuesdays, Thursdays, and Fridays, and four exercises for the back and biceps on both Wednesdays and Saturdays. Although players had their choice of exercise, they had to perform the following core exercises: bench press, squat, push press, power clean, and deadlift. Performance improvements as a percentage from baseline can be examined in Table 3.3.

All players in the study were experienced in resistance training with an average experience level of three years. Players in the three-day group were significantly weaker than all other groups in squat strength, while no differences were noted between the groups in bench press strength. The six-day per week training group were significantly slower than all other groups in the 40-yard sprint, and had significantly lower vertical jump power than the three-day group only. Results indicated that the five-day per week training group experienced significant increases in both bench press and squat strength, while the four- and six-day training groups realized significant gains in squat strength only. In the four- to six-day per week training groups, increases in 1RM strength ranged from 6.5% in the strongest group to 7.5%. Improvements in 1RM bench press ranged from 3.5% to 4% in four-, five-, and six-day per week groups. The players in the three-day per week group had the lowest percentage gains, despite being significantly weaker in the squat exercise than all other groups. No changes were noted in speed or vertical jump power. The investigators concluded that the five-day per week training group had the greatest impact on strength. It was also noted that the lack of strength gains in the three-day per week group may have been related to an insufficient use of assistance exercises, which may be important for experienced, resistance-trained athletes (Hoffman et al., 1990).

A later study that was also conducted at the University of Connecticut examined the effect of training experience in performance gains during a ten-week, nonlinear periodized off-season conditioning program (Smith et al., 2014). Players were grouped by years in the program as follows: first-year players were group 1, second- and third-year players were group 2, and fourth- and fifth-year players were group 3. Each training group had different training goals. Group 1 prioritized body mass gains, group 2 prioritized strength gains, and group 3 prioritized power gains. Prior to the training program, no significant differences were noted between the groups in body mass. However, significant differences were noted in 1RM bench press and 1RM squat between the groups, with group 3 being the strongest of the groups. The percent changes from baseline levels during this investigation are depicted in Table 3.3. No significant changes were noted in body mass in any of the groups. Significant increases in 1RM strength for both the bench press and squat exercises were reported in groups 1 and 2 only, but no changes were

TABLE 3.3 Performance Changes (%) During Off-Season Conditioning Programs for Football

Study (Athletes)	Study Duration	Training Frequency	1 RM Bench Press	1 RM Squat	40-yard Sprint	VJ Power	Body Mass
Hoffman et al., 1990 (n = 12,15,23,11, respectively) (Collegiate)	10 weeks	Three days	1.8	5.2	0.0	1.2	−0.9
		Four days	3.5	7.3*	0.8	0.2	−1.2*
		Five days	4.0*	7.5*	0.8	2.3	−0.5
		Six days	4.0	6.5*	1.0	4.3	−1.2
Bemben et al., 2001 (n = 8) (Collegiate)	9 weeks	Four days	0.2	5.0*	–	–	0.7
Wilder et al., 2001 (n = 9) (Collegiate)	10 weeks	Four days	–	5.3%	–	–	–
Hoffman et al., 2007 (n = 10) (Collegiate)	12 weeks	Four days	6.8*	6.9*	–	–	0.3
Smith et al., 2014 (n = 20/group) (Collegiate)	10 weeks	Four days			–		
		Group 1	3.4*	6.4*		− 1.5	1.3
		Group 2	4.0*	7.9*		1.9	0.9
		Group 3	0	− 0.3		− 2.9	1.1
Wroble and Moxley, 2001 (n = 39) (High School)	4 months	Three days	13.2*	13.8*	–	7.0*	5.5*

* = significantly different (p < 0.05)

noted in vertical jump power. These results highlight the principle of diminishing returns. The stronger and most experienced athletes experienced only limited gains in strength compared to the other, less experienced and weaker athletes.

The studies specifically examining the efficacy of off-season strength and conditioning programs are limited. To expand the data depicted in Table 3.3, studies that used off-season conditioning to examine various nutrients were added (Bemben et al., 2001; Hoffman et al., 2007; Wilder et al., 2001). These investigations generally used small data sets (subjects per group ranging from 8 to 10); thus, it is important to examine these results within the appropriate context.

An examination of high school football players participating in a four-month, three-day per week training program experienced significant improvements in both bench press and squat strength (see Table 3.3) (Wroble and Moxley, 2001). In addition, significant improvements were also noted in vertical jump height and body mass. However, the gain in body mass appeared to come primarily from increases in fat mass and not from lean mass gains. The authors compared these results to a group of football players who participated in the training program but also played a winter sport. Although strength gains were seen in both groups, the gains achieved by the conditioning only group were significantly greater.

Comparison of Different Modes of Training (Olympic Lifting and Ballistic Training) to Traditional Power Lifting During Off-Season Conditioning for Football

Most resistance training programs for football have traditionally used a power lifting program. In novice resistance-trained athletes, large increases in strength are common during the beginning stages of training. Improvements in various power components of athletic performance, such as vertical jump height and sprint speed, may also be evident (Hoffman, 2014). This is primarily the result of the athlete being able to generate a greater amount of force. As the athlete becomes stronger and more experienced, the rate of strength development decreases and eventually reaches a plateau. At this stage of the athlete's career, not only are strength improvements harder to achieve, but improving maximal strength may also not provide the same stimulus to power performance as it did during the earlier stages of training. In addition, training for maximum force development may have its limitations on improving power performance. An important factor for maximizing power production is exerting as much force as possible in a short period of time. By training for maximal strength through heavy resistance training, the rate of force development does not appear to be enhanced (Kraemer and Newton, 2000). The change in stimulus from a high force and low velocity to one of high force and high velocity may augment performance improvements in experienced, resistance-trained football players. The addition of plyometric and/or ballistic training may provide a greater stimulus for increasing the rate of force development.

The importance of exerting maximal force as rapidly as possible is the basis for success in strength/power sports (Hoffman, 2014). This is referred to as the maximum rate of force development (mRFD). The importance of mRFD is often seen in football. Success is often determined by who controls the line of scrimmage. Who would be victorious between two opposing players of similar size, strength, and technique? It would be the athlete who can reach maximal force faster. As the players slam into one another and attempt to extend their arms and control their opponent, the athlete who can generate maximal force quicker will have an advantage. By incorporating high-velocity movements into the athlete's training program, the rate of force development can be enhanced more so than focusing primarily on increasing maximal strength. Although the rate of force development is improved by heavy-resistance exercise, the magnitude of improvement is superior with higher velocity exercises (Hoffman, 2014).

The goal of enhancing power performance has been the basis for the inclusion of Olympic-style lifts in the training program of football players. For many years, coaches have employed Olympic lifting exercises in the training program of football players, but their efficacy in comparison to the traditional power lifting exercises were largely unknown. Despite the widespread acceptance of Olympic lifting exercises as part of the resistance training program of football players, there has been limited evidence to support the large popularity of this mode of training. The first study to compare Olympic and traditional power lifting training was conducted in NCAA Division III football players during their off-season conditioning program (Hoffman et al., 2004a). Twenty players were assigned to either an Olympic weight lifting or power lifting group. Each group was matched for football position. Subjects were assigned to the Olympic weight lifting group based upon their competency in the techniques demonstrated in previous training programs performed at the college. Both training programs were performed four-days per week for 15 weeks. The preparatory phase of the training program was five weeks in duration and was similar for both groups. During the strength phase of training (weeks 6–10), each group began their specific training program. For the next two phases, each lasting five weeks, players performed their group-specific training program. The only similarity between the training programs was the bench press and squat exercises, which were maintained at similar training volume and intensities, since both of these exercises were part of the athletes testing program. Subjects were provided a range of repetitions to perform at a recommended intensity of their 1RM for each exercise. Table 3.4 provides the training programs for both the Olympic and

TABLE 3.4 Olympic and Power Lifting Training Program Comparisons

Preparatory Phase		Strength Phase		Strength/Power Phase	
Both Groups		Olympic Lifting Group		Olympic Lifting Group	
Monday and Thursday	Tuesday and Friday	Monday	Thursday	Monday	Thursday
Bench Press 4 × 8–10 RM	Squats 4 × 8–10 RM	Snatch (above knee) 5 × 5 RM	Snatch (floor) 5 × 5 RM	Snatch (floor) 5 × 3 RM	Clean (above knee) 5 × 3 RM
Incline bench press 3 × 8–10 RM	Dead Lift 4 × 8–10 RM	Snatch Pull (floor) 5 × 5 RM	Snatch Pull (waist) 5 × 5 RM	Push Jerks 5 × 3 RM	Squats 5 × 4–6 RM
Dumbbell incline Fly's 3 × 8–10 RM	Leg extensions 3 × 8–10 RM	Bench press 4 × 6–8 RM	Push jerk 5 × 5 RM	Squats 5 × 4–6 RM	Jump squats (30% 1RM) 4 × 5 RM
Seated shoulder press 4 × 8–10 RM	Leg curls 3 × 8–10 RM	Dumbbell pulls (floor) 5 × 5 RM	Bench press 4 × 6–8 RM	Box jumps 3 × 8	Dumbbell push press 4 × 3 RM
Upright rows 3 × 8–10 RM	Standing calf raises 3 × 8–10 RM	Push press 5 × 5 RM	Front squat 5 × 6–8 RM	Lunges 3 × 6–8 RM	Snatch pulls (waist) 3 × 3 RM
Lateral raises 3 × 8–10 RM	Lateral pulldowns 4 × 8–10 RM	*Tuesday*	*Friday*	*Tuesday*	*Friday*
Triceps pushdowns 3 × 8–10 RM	Seated row 4 × 8–10 RM	Clean (floor) 5 × 5 RM	Clean (above knee) 5 × 5 RM	Overhead squats 4 × 6–8 RM	Clean pulls (waist) 3 × 3 RM
Triceps extension 3 × 8–10 RM	Biceps curls 4 × 8–10 RM	Clean pull (above knee) 5 × 5 RM	Dumbbell push press 5 × 5 RM	Snatch (floor) 5 × 3 RM	Front squats 3 × 5 RM

Preparatory Phase		Strength Phase		Strength/Power Phase	
Both Groups		Olympic Lifting Group		Olympic Lifting Group	
Monday and Thursday	Tuesday and Friday	Monday	Thursday	Monday	Thursday
Sit-ups	Sit-ups	Push jerks 5 × 5 RM	Squats 4 × 6–8 RM	Clean pulls (above knee) 3 × 5 RM	Box jumps with dumbbell 3 × 5
		Squats 4 × 6–8 RM	Power shrugs 5 × 5 RM	Bench press 5 × 4–6 RM	Bench press 5 × 4–6 RM
		Lunges 4 × 6–8 RM	Overhead squats 4 × 6–8 RM	Push press 5 × 3 RM	Power shrugs 5 × 5 RM
		Power Lifting Group			
		Monday	Thursday	Monday	Thursday
		Squats 4 × 6–8 RM	Squats 4 × 6–8 RM	Squats 5 × 4–6 RM	Squats 5 × 4–6 RM
		Dead lift 3 × 6–8 RM[1]	Stiff leg dead lift 3 × 6–8 RM	Dead lift 4 × 4–6 RM	Romanian dead lift 4 × 4–6 RM
		Leg curl 3 × 6–8 RM	Leg curl 3 × 6–8 RM	Leg curl 3 × 4–6 RM	Leg curl 3 × 4–6 RM
		Standing calf raise 3 × 6–8 RM	Standing calf raise 3 × 6–8 RM	Standing calf raise 3 × 4–6 RM	Standing calf raise 3 × 4–6 RM
		Lateral pulldown 4 × 6–8 RM	Lateral pulldown 4 × 6–8 RM	Lateral pulldown 5 × 4–6 RM	Lateral pulldown 5 × 4–6 RM
		Seated row 4 × 6–8 RM	Seated row 4 × 6–8 RM	Seated row 5 × 4–6 RM	Seated row 5 × 4–6 RM
		Biceps curl 4 × 6–8 RM	Biceps curl 4 × 6–8 RM	Biceps curl 4 × 4–6 RM	Biceps curl 4 × 4–6 RM
		Sit-ups	Sit-ups	Sit-ups	Sit-ups
		Tuesday	Friday	Tuesday	Friday
		Bench press 4 × 6–8 RM	Bench press 4 × 6–8 RM	Bench press 5 × 4–6 RM	Bench press 5 × 4–6 RM
		Incline dumbbell bench press 4 × 6–8 RM	Incline bench press close grip 4 × 6–8 RM	Incline dumbbell bench press 5 × 4–6 RM[2]	Incline bench press close grip 4 × 6–8 RM
		Incline flys (flat bench) 3 × 6–8 RM	Incline flys (flat bench) 3 × 6–8 RM	Seated dumbbell shoulder press 5 × 4–6 RM	Seated dumbbell shoulder press 5 × 4–6 RM
		Seated dumbbell shoulder press 4 × 6–8 RM	Seated dumbbell shoulder press 4 × 6–8 RM	Upright row 4 × 4–6 RM	Upright row 4 × 4–6 RM
		Upright row 3 × 6–8 RM	Upright row 3 × 6–8 RM	Triceps extension 4 × 4–6 RM	Triceps pushdown 4 × 4–6 RM
		Front raise 3 × 6–8 RM	Lateral raise 3 × 6–8 RM	Sit-ups	Sit-ups
		Triceps extension 4 × 6–8 RM	Triceps pushdown 4 × 6–8 RM		
		Sit-ups	Sit-ups		

Source: Hoffman et al., 2004a.

Note: RM = Repetition maximum.

power lifting groups. In addition to the resistance training program, all players participated in a two-day per week sprint and agility training program. This program was performed during the strength/power phase of the training program, and it was required for all members of the football team, including those participating in the study.

No between-group differences in 1RM bench press and 1RM squat strength were observed between the groups. In addition, no significant change was observed in the 1RM bench press in either the Olympic lifting (4.4%) or power lifting (9.6%) groups, but significant improvements were noted in 1RM squat (12.9% and 12.8%, respectively, for both groups). No significant changes in body mass were noted in either the Olympic lifting (0.8% increase) or the power lifting (0.3% increase) group. Interestingly, the Olympic lifting group had a significantly greater improvement in vertical jump height (5.9%) than the power lifting group (−0.7%). In addition, 40-yard sprint time was reduced in the Olympic lifting group by −1.4%, and by only −0.8% in the power lifting group. Although these differences were not statistically different, the improvements in 40-yard sprint times were 175% greater in the Olympic lifting group compared to the power lifting group (0.07 ± 0.14 s compared to 0.04 ± 0.11 s, respectively). Results of this investigation suggest that an Olympic weight lifting program may provide a greater advantage in improving vertical jump performance than traditional power lifting. In addition, trends seen in 40-yard sprint speed suggested that the sprint and agility training program, performed during the strength/power phase of training in both groups, was a confounding factor that likely affected some of the results observed.

There have been only two other investigations known that have compared Olympic and power lifting training programs in football players. This is a bit surprising considering the importance that is placed on power development in strength/power athletes (Haff, 2001). Channell and Barfield (2008) examined the effect of Olympic and traditional resistance training on vertical jump improvements in high school football players. In this eight-week study, the investigators reported significant improvements in vertical jump performance in both the Olympic (2.46 ± 4.7 cm) and power lifting programs (1.16 ± 3.1 cm). The changes in vertical jump performance represented a 4.5% increase for the Olympic lifting group and a 2.3% increase in the power lifting group. These results were similar to that previously reported by Hoffman et al. (2004a). A subsequent study also examined high school football players performing Olympic lifting or traditional power lifting for eight weeks (Roberts and DeBeliso, 2018). The investigators reported significantly greater improvements in 1RM squat in the Olympic lifting group (17.2% increase) compared to the players participating in the traditional power lifting program (10.6%). Although both groups improved vertical jump performance, no differences were noted between the Olympic lifting (5.3%) and traditional power lifting (5.1%) groups. In addition, no changes were noted in 9.1 m sprint speed. Interestingly, the studies comparing Olympic to traditional power lifting training programs have not been overwhelmingly positive. Although positive trends regarding greater improvements have been noted in lower body strength, speed, and power, these changes have not been statistically convincing. However, it should be acknowledged that small differences may take on a greater magnitude in sports in which success often hinges on a difference of a fraction of a second.

Ballistic training is another training mode that is used to enhance the rate of force development (Kraemer and Newton, 2000). Ballistic exercises such as jump squats, bench press throws, or medicine ball throws allow the athlete to accelerate a force through a complete range of motion. One study examined the effect of adding a jump squat to the training program of competitive football players during the power phase of the off-season conditioning program (Hoffman et al., 2005a). Forty-seven experienced, resistance-trained football players competing at a NCAA Division III institution were assigned to either a group that performed the jump squat exercise with both concentric and eccentric phases of movement, a group that performed the jump squat exercise using only the concentric phase of movement, or a control group (players who did not perform the jump squat exercise) during the team's off-season strength and conditioning program. The squat jump was performed on a device that had the option of unloading the eccentric phase of the jump. Unloading was accomplished via a hydraulic system that was able to catch the bar after it reached its peak height. All squat jumps were performed using 70% of the athlete's 1RM squat. The athletes performed the exercise using shoulder pads to exert effort. No bar was placed across the athletes cervical vertebrae. All groups performed the identical off-season strength and conditioning program. The jump squat exercise was included in the strength/power phase (five weeks) of the athletes' off-season periodized training program. Strength, power, speed, and agility were measured prior to and following the off-season training program. Significant differences were seen in the change (Δ) in 1RM squat and Δ1RM power clean between the jump squat group that used both concentric and eccentric phases of the jump movement compared to the control group. No other between-group differences were seen in these variables, and no significant differences were seen between the groups in Δ speed, Δ agility, and Δ vertical jump height. Although the jump squat was performed on a jump squat machine, the relatively high intensity used for training may have been a disadvantage in stimulating power gains by minimizing velocity of movement compared to lower intensities of training. In addition, a short-duration training program may not have been sufficient to elicit significant changes in an experienced, trained group of athletes. No other studies are known that have specifically examined the effects of ballistic training in competitive football players during any part of the yearly training cycle.

Efficacy of Inseason Strength and Conditioning Programs for Football

The goal of the off-season conditioning programs is to enhance the athletes' potential for success during the season. If the training stimulus is removed, the athlete's ability to maintain strength and power gains would be compromised. This is the basis of the principle of reversibility. During the inseason training program, the primary emphasis is on football practices. However, to maintain the gains made in the off-season, coaches have to maintain a training stimulus. They generally reduce intensity of training to about 80% of the maximum 1RM and also decrease the frequency and volume of training (Hoffman, 2014). The inseason training program generally consists of performing the core exercises twice per week. There have been only a few studies that have examined the effectiveness of inseason training program. Hoffman and Kang (2003) required football players from a NCAA Division III program to perform the power clean (1,3 × 3–5 RM), squat (1,3 × 6–8 RM), push press (1,3 × 4–6 RM), and bench press (1,3 × 6–8 RM) exercises twice per week. All players performed at least one warm-up set and then three sets with a load that allowed them to achieve the required RM. There was 72 h between each training session. The inseason training program began during the preseason and lasted the entire competitive season. Results of the study indicated that football players were able to maintain both their upper and lower body strength during the competitive season, while using a two-day per week maintenance program, with loads equating to 80% of the athletes' 1RM during each training session. An interesting outcome of the study revealed that when training intensity exceeded 80% of the players 1RM, the ability to stimulate strength improvements is significantly greater than when training intensity was below 80%, especially in first-year players. It was suggested that the accumulated fatigue occurring in players who have greater playing time likely limits the extent of muscle adaptation during the season. Interestingly, the intensity of exercise was significantly correlated to the change in both 1RM bench press ($r = 0.68$, $p < 0.05$) and 1RM squat ($r = 0.47$, $p < 0.05$).

Another study from the same research group examined two types of inseason training programs in freshman football players (Hoffman et al., 2003). One program was the traditional linear program in which both workouts of the week were identical and the other program was nonlinear. In the nonlinear program, the exercises were the same, but the intensity and volume of training were different for each workout of the week. The first workout of the week required the subjects to perform three sets at either four to six repetitions (power clean and push press) or eight to ten repetitions (bench press and squat) at 70% of 1RM. The second workout of the week required the players to perform two to four repetitions for three sets for all exercises at 90% of 1RM. Results of the study revealed a significant improvement during the season in the 1RM squat in the linear model but not in the nonlinear model. No significant improvements in the 1RM bench press or in the body mass were noted in either group. The results of these investigations suggested that intensity of training in an inseason maintenance program needs to be at least 80% of 1RM to maintain strength in experienced, resistance-trained football players or stimulate strength improvements in players with limited resistance training experience.

Comparison of Various Periodization Paradigms in Football

The goal of periodized training programs is to manipulate both training intensity and training volume to help the athlete reach peak condition prior to the start of competition (Hoffman, 2014). The concept of periodization primarily came out of the development of year-long or multi-year training programs for weight lifters competing in international competitions (Matveev, 1958). In 1981, Dr. Mike Stone adapted many of these concepts and suggested that it could be applied to the training program of American football players (Stone et al., 1981). Most investigations examining various periodization schemes have not been performed on competitive athletes. Even fewer studies have compared different periodization models to no periodization. Many of the studies that have examined different training modalities or interventions often use a periodized training routine. The duration of the study is often less than 15 weeks in duration. The reason for this study duration is that it fits into the academic semester. Even in the optimal situation, a 15-week periodized training program was not the basis for why periodization programming was developed. Thus, the question of whether a 15-week off-season resistance training program in football players is efficacious compared to no periodization scheme is a legitimate question. Does manipulation of intensity and volume of training effective in a relatively short time period provide any advantage?

Part of the problem in examining this question includes a number of logistical and practical issues. Most athletic teams do not have the roster numbers to provide sufficient statistical power for an extended study examining various training paradigms. This limits the potential to conduct research studies in football players. This requires a tremendous degree of cooperation that unfortunately doesn't always exist. Despite having limited evidence supporting the use of a periodization model for training strength/power athletes, including football players, the concept of periodization has gained widespread acceptance (Issurin, 2016; Mujika et al., 2018; Williams et al., 2017).

The first study to examine the efficacy of periodization in college football players was published in 2009 (Hoffman et al., 2009a). The purpose of the study was to compare two primary periodization schemes (linear and nonlinear) to a no periodization program in NCAA Division III college football players. A common characteristic of conditioning programs in Division III collegiate athletes is a relatively long active rest period between the conclusion of the season and the onset of the off-season training program. Thus, it was important to interpret the results of the study with that important context in mind. Fifty-one experienced, resistance-trained players were randomly assigned to one of three groups that differed only in the manipulation of intensity and volume of training during the four-day per week, split routine, 15-week spring semester off-season resistance training program. A one-week off period occurred after week 7 for spring break. Testing occurred at weeks 0 (pre), 7 (mid), and 15 (post). One group of athletes performed the same training program for the entire study (6–8 RM in traditional power exercises and 3–4 RM in Olympic movement exercises). This was considered the no periodization (NP) group. Another group of athletes were randomized into a linear periodization (LP) group in which they did a four-week hypertrophy (9–12 RM) phase, six-week strength phase (6–8 RM in power lifting exercises and 3–4 RM in Olympic movement exercises), and a four-week power phase (3–5 RM in power lifting exercises and 1–2 RM in the Olympic movement exercises). The final group was a nonlinear periodization group (NLP). They performed a power phase (3–5 RM) twice per week and a hypertrophy phase (9–12 RM) the other two days of the week for the entire training study. The percent changes in strength performance can be observed in Figure 3.3. Significant increases were seen in all three groups in both the 1RM bench press and 1RM squat. However, no differences in the magnitude of improvement were noted between the groups. The greatest increases though were observed in the first seven weeks of training in all three groups. Interestingly, the NLP group experienced no further increase (0.1%) from mid- to post-testing for squat strength. The large increase in strength in the first seven weeks of the training program likely reflects the long detraining period that occurred between the end of the season and the start of the off-season conditioning program. Similar results were also seen in vertical jump performance. Significant improvements were noted in NP (4.1%), LP (2.4%), and NLP (3.2%) between pre to mid. However, no other changes were noted. Thus, during a short-duration training program (~14 weeks), the benefits of a periodized

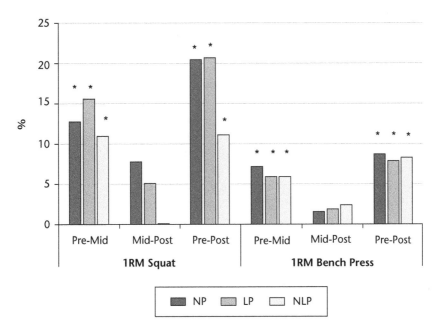

FIGURE 3.3   Comparison of Linear Periodization, Nonlinear Periodization, and No Periodization in Maximal Upper and Lower Body Strength in an Off-Season Conditioning Program for Football. NP = no periodization; LP = linear periodization; NLP = nonlinear periodization; ★ = significant increase. All data are reported as % increase.

Source: Data from Hoffman et al., 2009a.

training program may not be realized. Again, it is important to understand that training programs are developed for the entire year. Thus, the benefits of a periodized training program are likely more relevant in having the athlete peak at the appropriate time of the year and minimize the risk of overtraining. However, periodization may not directly be associated with maximal performance development. This is the only investigation that has been conducted on periodization programs in football players. The results do not support the benefits of periodizing the training program, but coaches and sport scientists who work with these athletes do need to monitor their athletes to ensure appropriate loading, which is challenging but provides adequate recovery.

Physical Performance Changes in the Football Player's Career

There are only a limited number of studies that have examined physical and performance changes in high school football players. A recent study indicated that a maturation process is seen in these players with the largest changes in performance occurring between the 10th and 11th grades (Dupler et al., 2010). This appears to be consistent across offensive and defensive players. Consideration for adjusting rosters (e.g., varsity versus junior varsity teams) to account for athlete maturation may provide a method of not pushing or rushing athletes before they are physically ready for the next level of competition.

Anzell and colleagues (2011) examined changes in height, body mass, and body composition in both collegiate and professional football players over several decades. They reported a significant increase in body mass for collegiate (linemen and skill position players) and professional football players (linemen and offensive backs) over time. The investigators also reported a significant increase in percent body fat in college football players (all positions combined) but not in professional players. No changes were observed in body height, in either collegiate or professional players. A similar examination, albeit in Division III college football players who participated in New England schools between 1956 and 2014, reported significant changes in body mass over the 50+years examined (Elliott et al., 2016). Increases in body mass ranged from 5.7% in wide receivers to 37.5% in offensive linemen. Significant increases in height were also seen over time in linemen, tight ends, defensive ends, and quarterbacks. No changes in height were noted in any of the other positions. Changes in height ranged from 1.1% in linebackers to 3.8% in offensive linemen. Others have looked at changes in anthropometry over a much shorter duration. In a study of NCAA Division I football players, Trexler and colleagues (2017) examined 57 football players during a single year and a smaller subset (n = 13) during their four-year collegiate career. Using dual-energy X-ray absorptiometry (DEXA), measurements were taken on four occasions – beginning and end of the off-season (March–May), preseason (mid-July), and the start of the following off-season (March). Significant increases in lean mass were noted from the end of the off-season to the preseason period, and a greater change was noted from the preseason to the start of the following off-season period. Both bone mineral content and bone mineral density increased over time. In addition, significant reductions were also reported for body fat percentage and fat mass. Examination of changes over the player's career indicated that body mass significantly increased between years 1 and 2 and between years 2 and 3. No significant change was noted between the players third and fourth years of eligibility. Weight gain over the four-year career was slightly greater in linemen compared to skill position players (8.5 ± 5.4 kg and 5.4 ± 2.7 kg, respectively). Lean mass was significantly greater in the athletes' fourth year (83.7 ± 8.2 kg) than the previous three seasons (79.4 ± 7.4 kg, 80.6 ± 7.1 kg, and 80.6 ± 7.8 kg, respectively). Lean mass changes over the players' career were also greater in linemen

(6.2 ± 3.2 kg) than skill position players (3.1 ± 2.4 kg). No significant changes were noted in body fat composition or fat mass during the four-year career.

Several studies have examined performance changes in the careers of college football players. A study in NCAA Division I football players reported significant gains in body mass, lean body mass, number of repetitions performed with the 102 kg bench press test, agility, and vertical jump height (Stodden and Galitski, 2010). The investigators reported that during the athletes' four-year career, body mass increased every year but the fourth year. Body mass increased 2.2% for all positions combined from the first to third year, but decreased 1.5% from year 3 to year 4. These results were less than those subsequently reported in both NCAA Division I and Division III players (Hoffman et al., 2011; Jacobson et al., 2013). Table 3.5 compares body mass changes in the four-year career of college football players separated by position. Body mass increased 5.9% during the four-year career of NCAA Division III players (6.1% in linemen and 4.9% in skill position players). Interestingly, NCAA Division I linemen only gained 2.9% body mass during their career, whereas skill position players increased their body mass by 9.0%. The lower body mass gains seen in the Division I linemen compared to the Division III linemen reflect the large difference in body mass seen in the athletes first year of competition. Body size is likely one of the discriminating factors separating Division I and Division III football players. The Division I players were bigger (~23 kg) as freshman, which likely contributed to them being a scholarship athlete compared to the non-scholarship Division III player.

Changes in strength during a four-year career in Division I and Division III football players are depicted in Table 3.6. Improvements in 1RM bench press during a college career in football players have been reported to range between 17.7% and 34.1% (Hoffman et al., 2011; Jacobson et al., 2013; Miller et al., 2002). Improvements in upper body strength among linemen appear to be greater in the Division III players (22.7%) than the Division I players (17.8%). However, Division I skill position players experienced a nearly threefold greater improvement in upper body strength than Division III skill position players (34.1% versus 12.5%, respectively). Similar improvements in squat strength were noted between Division I and Division III linemen (27.4% and 25.6%, respectively), but Division I skill position players had a twofold greater increase (32.4%) in squat strength than Division III skill position players (15.8%). Interestingly, the average

TABLE 3.5 Body Mass Changes in a Four-Year Career in NCAA Division I and III College Football Players

	League and Players	Year 1	Year 2	% Change	Year 3	% Change	Year 4	% Change	Total % Change
Body mass (kg)	DIII All players	93.7 ± 17.1	95.2 ± 16.7	1.6	97.4 ± 17.1	2.3	99.2 ± 18.6	1.8^	5.9#
	DIII Linemen	105.8 ± 15.3	108.0 ± 14.9	2.1	109.5 ± 14.7	1.4	112.3 ± 15.8	2.6^	6.1#
	DIII Skill positions	81.8 ± 8.3	84.2 ± 8.1	2.9*	85.4 ± 8.9	1.4	85.8 ± 9.3	0.5	4.9#
	D1 Linemen	128.7 ± 12.7	131.2 ± 10.8	1.9*	131.9 ± 8.5	0.5	132.4 ± 8.2	0.4	2.9#
	D1 DB and WR	79.7 ± 7.5	85.8 ± 8.8	7.7*	84.6 ± 8.5	−1.4	86.9 ± 5.7	2.7	9.0#

Source: Data from Hoffman et al., 2011 (NCAA DIII) and Jacobson et al., 2013 (NCAA DI).

Notes: All data are reported as mean ± SD. * = significantly different from previous year; ^ = significantly different from year 1; # = significant improvement in career; DB = defensive backs; WR = wide receivers.

TABLE 3.6 Strength Performance Changes in a Four-Year Career in NCAA Division I and III College Football Players

	League and Players	Year 1	Year 2	% Change	Year 3	% Change	Year 4	% Change	Total % Change
Bench press (kg)	DIII All players	117.4 ± 20.9	126.7 ± 20.4	7.9*	134.5 ± 21.7	6.2*	138.2 ± 21.9	2.8	17.7#
	DIII Linemen	122.7 ± 20.9	132.2 ± 19.7	7.7★	143.1 ± 20.5	8.2*	150.6 ± 20.0	5.2	22.7#
	DIII Skill positions	112.3 ± 19.1	121.8 ± 19.8	8.4*	125.7 ± 19.3	3.2*	126.3 ± 19.4	0.5	12.5#
	D1 Linemen	159.3 ± 23.6	171.2 ± 17.9	7.7*	181.8 ± 18.7	6.2*	187.7 ± 19.0	3.3	17.8#
	D1 DB and WR	105.5 ± 17.6	125.8 ± 15.2	19.2*	135.5 ± 17.7	7.7	141.5 ± 7.7	4.4	34.1#
Squat (kg)	DIII All players	152.5 ± 27.3	166.4 ± 28.4	9.1*	179.8 ± 30.4	8.1*	184.8 ± 33.7	2.8	21.2#
	DIII Linemen	157.7 ± 28.5	168.6 ± 28.5	6.9*	188.4 ± 29.1	11.7*	198.0 ± 32.3	5.1	25.6#
	DIII Skill positions	147.3 ± 25.0	164.4 ± 28.3	11.6*	170.0 ± 29.2	3.4	170.6 ± 29.4	0.4	15.8#
	D1 Linemen	210.0 ± 33.8	242.8 ± 32.4	15.6*	258.6 ± 26.8	6.5*	267.6 ± 33.6	3.3	27.4#
	D1 DB and WR	155.2 ± 28.0	180.0 ± 26.2	15.8*	196.5 ± 21.6	9.1*	205.5 ± 16.2	4.6	32.4#

Source: Data from Hoffman et al., 2011 (NCAA DIII) and Jacobson et al., 2013 (NCAA DI).

Notes: All data are reported as mean ± SD. * = significantly different from previous year; # = significant improvement in career; DB = defensive backs; WR = wide receivers.

squat strength of Division I skill position players was similar to or greater than that seen in Division III linemen. The ability of strength performance to differentiate between different levels of play will be discussed in further detail in Chapter 4. Examination of year-to-year strength improvements indicated that the greatest gains in strength occurred during the athlete's freshman year (year 1). Significant strength gains were also reported during the sophomore off-season (between years 2 and 3) in all Division I athletes, but only linemen at the Division III level. Skill position players for Division III football experienced significant strength gains in both the bench press and squat exercises only following the freshman off-season. These differences in the magnitude of strength gains among skill position athletes in the two divisions of play are not clear, but it may be related to the size of the strength and conditioning staffs and access to training tables common in Division I programs that do not occur at the Division III level. Considering that the skill position players have a much greater window of strength adaptation available to them, external factors such as facility, personnel, and nutrition may have all contributed to these differences.

Table 3.7 depicts changes in 40-yard sprint speed and vertical jump height in the career of Division I and III football players. Significant improvements were noted in Division III players (both linemen and skill position players) in vertical jump height (Hoffman et al., 2011). However, in contrast to strength performance, significant changes in vertical jump height (a measure of lower body power) took longer to achieve. Significant gains were not seen until the athlete's senior year. This may reflect a greater emphasis on power training in these older athletes. These results were consistent with other longitudinal studies examining collegiate football (Miller et al., 2002). No changes in vertical jump height were noted in the four-year career of Division I

TABLE 3.7 Speed and Jump Performance Changes in a Four-Year Career in NCAA Division I and III College Football Players

	League and Players	Year 1	Year 2	% Change	Year 3	% Change	Year 4	% Change	Total % Change
40-yard Sprint (s)	DIII All players	5.05 ± 0.34	5.01 ± 0.37	−0.8	4.97 ± 0.37	−0.8	4.95 ± 0.35	−0.4	−2.0
	DIII Linemen	5.24 ± 0.35	5.23 ± 0.38	−0.2	5.18 ± 0.37	−1.0	5.13 ± 0.37	−1.0	−2.1
	DIII Skill positions	4.86 ± 0.20	4.81 ± 0.21	−1.0	4.77 ± 0.23	−0.8^	4.77 ± 0.20	0	−1.9#
	D1 Linemen	5.36 ± 0.23	5.29 ± 0.23	−1.3	5.17 ± 0.22	−2.3	5.17 ± 0.19	0	−3.5
	D1 DB and WR	4.58 ± 0.16	4.53 ± 0.11	−1.1	4.53 ± 0.16	0	4.50 ± 0.10	−0.7	−1.7
Vertical jump height (cm)	DIII All players	64.9 ± 9.5	66.5 ± 9.2	2.5	66.4 ± 9.0	0	69.7 ± 9.8	5.0*	7.4#
	DIII Linemen	61.0 ± 10.1	62.6 ± 8.4	2.6	63.6 ± 9.2	1.6	66.3 ± 9.5	4.2^*	8.7#
	DIII Skill positions	68.4 ± 7.5	69.8 ± 8.5	2.0	69.6 ± 7.7	−0.3	73.4 ± 8.9	5.5^	7.3#
	D1 Linemen	65.5 ± 7.1	64.8 ± 7.6	−1.1	67.1 ± 7.9	3.5	67.3 ± 6.6	0.3	2.7
	D1 DB and WR	83.1 ± 5.8	86.9 ± 6.6	4.6*	88.9 ± 6.4	2.3	89.9 ± 6.1	1.1	8.2#

Source: Data from Hoffman et al., 2011 (NCAA DIII) and Jacobson et al., 2013 (NCAA DI).

Notes: All data are reported as mean ± SD. * = significantly different from previous year; ^ = significantly different from year 1; # = significant improvement in career; DB = defensive backs; WR = wide receivers.

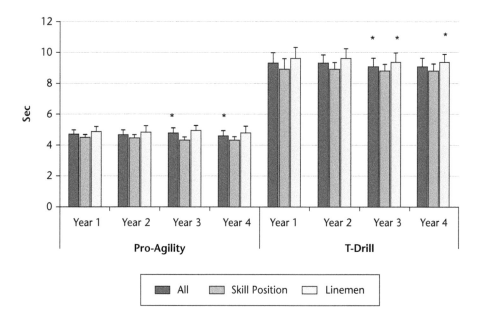

FIGURE 3.4   Changes in Agility Performance in Division III College Football Players.

* = significantly different from year 1. All data are reported as mean ± SD.

Source: Data from Hoffman et al., 2011.

college linemen, but a significant change was seen in Division I skill position players (Jacobson et al., 2013). The largest gains were noted in the athletes' freshman year. This is consistent with the improvements seen in strength. It is likely that the greatest physical trait that separated the Division I skill position players from the Division III players was speed. Their greatest window of opportunity was actually in improving strength. Thus, the significant strength improvement in lower body strength in these athletes during their freshman year had a greater impact on power performance. Keep in mind that power is defined as force × velocity. As velocity was already at a high level, it was the force potential that had the greatest window of growth.

The ability to improve speed and agility appears to be limited. If speed is improved, it generally occurs during the later stages of the athlete's playing career (Hoffman et al., 2011; Jacobson et al., 2013). Division III athletes appeared to decrease 0.1 s from their 40-yard sprint time during their four-year career, while Division I skill position players were slightly less (0.08 s) and linemen almost twice as much (0.19 s). It is likely that these performance variables are a function of genetic factors that impact the athletic potential of all athletes. Similar results were also noted in agility improvements. A nonsignificant 0.11 s decrease in time was noted in agility time (pro-agility test), but a significant improvement in time for the T-drill (0.22 s from freshman to junior seasons) in Division III football players (Hoffman et al., 2011) (see Figure 3.4).

Summary

To maximize the benefit of off-season conditioning programs, the strength and conditioning professional needs to understand the basic principles of training and develop scientifically sound training programs. It becomes imperative that strength and conditioning professionals are able to set appropriate training expectations and provide the correct exercises and loading schemes that maximize physiological adaptation from training. Most strength gains are observed during the early part of the athletes' career, while speed and agility improvements may take longer to develop. One of the more interesting issues related to the development of the yearly training program is the necessity of manipulating training intensity and training volume. Limited evidence suggests that there is no advantage in periodized training programs during a 15-week off-season training program.

4

PLAYER SELECTION AND PHYSICAL ATTRIBUTES FOR FOOTBALL PLAYING SUCCESS

Introduction

During the 2019 football season, the National Football League (NFL) celebrated its 100th anniversary. However, the first game of football is thought to have been played on November 6, 1869, between Princeton University and Rutgers University. Of the 150 years that football has been played, the importance of strength and conditioning has only been realized since the 1970s. Prior to that, most football coaches preferred that their players not lift weights for fear of becoming too "muscle bound" (Todd, 1992). Weight lifting started becoming popular in the 1960s, but most football players who lifted weights did so on their own and not under the guidance of a coach or a team (Shurley and Todd, 2012). It wasn't until the late 1960s that resistance training became an important part of preparation for football players. The strength and conditioning profession was born in the sport of football at the University of Nebraska. Boyd Epley, a student-athlete in track and field for the University of Nebraska, was asked to develop a strength program for the football team in 1969. He subsequently became the first strength coach in the United States. His success with the Cornhuskers led to other schools hiring coaches to develop the strength and conditioning programs. By 1978, Coach Epley reached out to these other coaches and 75 of them got together in Lincoln, Nebraska, to develop an organization called the National Strength and Conditioning Association (NSCA) (Shurley et al., 2017). Today the NSCA has nearly 30,000 members and just fewer than 56,000 individuals hold one of their strength and conditioning certifications. The motto of the NSCA is to bridge the gap between the science and the practitioner. There has not been a better organization in the world that has been able to create an opportunity for the top sport scientists to collaborate with coaches that are on the front lines of training competitive athletes. The past 40+ years has seen a tremendous growth in the strength and conditioning profession, but, more importantly, it has demonstrated the importance of strength, speed, and size on success in football, and has allowed coaches to gain a better understanding of the type of athletes who would be successful in the sport of football. This chapter will focus on the science of player selection and the physical attributes necessary to play the game of football.

Strength, Power, and Speed Comparisons Between Positions, Starters and Non-Starters, and Different Divisions of Play in College Football

Early studies examining the importance of strength, power, and speed identified that greater performance in these attributes contributed to football playing success (Barker et al., 1993; Berg et al., 1990; Black and Roundy, 1994; Fry and Kraemer, 1991). This understanding contributed to the growth of the strength coaching profession, and a greater emphasis placed on strength and conditioning programs at all levels of football (Hoffman, 2008; Kraemer and Gotshalk, 2000). An examination of the physical changes in football players from 1987 to 2000 indicated significant increases in the strength, power, and speed of players over that time span (Secora et al., 2004).

In 1987, one of the first studies to have published normative values appeared in the NSCA journal (Mayhew et al., 1987). This study compared linemen and skill position players on strength, speed, and power measures in National Collegiate Athletic Association (NCAA) Division II college football players. The investigators combined the results of three different college football teams playing in the same level of competition. The results indicated that linemen were taller, heavier, and stronger than the skill position players in the bench press, squat, and power clean exercises, but ran the 40-yard sprint slower and jumped lower than the skill position players. The strength and speed/power results of this study and others that made similar comparisons are depicted in Tables 4.1 and 4.2, respectively.

In 1991, Fry and Kraemer requested the preseason testing data from 30 collegiate strength and conditioning coaches from NCAA Division I, II, and III programs, with each category representing a balanced geographical cross section of the United States. Nineteen surveys were returned (Division I, n = 6; Division II, n = 7; Division III, n = 6) and the performance results of 981 players from the 1987 season were compared (Fry and Kraemer, 1991). Division I football players were significantly stronger than Division III players in the bench press and squat exercise and Division II and III players in the power clean exercise (see Table 4.1). Division I players were also faster than Division III players, and jumped significantly higher than players in both Division II and Division III (see Table 4.2). Comparisons in strength and speed performance between starters and nonstarters from the different divisions of college football by position can be seen in Tables 4.3 and 4.4, respectively. With playing divisions combined, significant differences were

TABLE 4.1 Strength Comparisons Between Linemen and Skill Position Players in College Football Players

Reference	NCAA Division	1RM Bench Press (kg)		1RM Squat (kg)		1RM Power Clean (kg)	
		Linemen	Skill	Linemen	Skill	Linemen	Skill
Mayhew et al., 1987	II	126.8 ± 22.3*	115.0 ± 22.3	179.1 ± 43.2*	165.9 ± 29.5	102.3 ± 13.2*	108.6 ± 14.5
Fry and	I	144.5 ± 26.1#		192.6 ± 37.6#		123.0 ± 17.9^	
Kraemer, 1991	II	135.2 ± 25.5		182.5 ± 34.4		116.5 ± 17.3	
	III	125.6 ± 23.2		176.9 ± 32.4		113.0 ± 16.5	
Schmidt, 1999	III	143.9 ± 22.3*	120.7 ± 20.0	–	–	–	–
Garstecki et al.,	I	165.0 ± 26.9*		231.6 ± 40.8*		138.6 ± 18.6*	
2004	II	145.8 ± 25.9		203.9 ± 41.2		126.2 ± 21.1	

Notes: 1RM = one repetition maximum. * = significantly different; # = significantly different than Division III only; ^ = significantly different than Division II and Division III. All data are reported as mean ± SD. One result indicates linemen and skill position players were combined.

TABLE 4.2 Speed and Vertical Jump Comparisons Between Linemen and Skill Position Players in College Football Players

Reference	NCAA Division	40-yard Sprint (s)		Vertical Jump (cm)	
		Linemen	Skill	Linemen	Skill
Mayhew et al., 1987	II	5.22 ± 0.26	4.91 ± 0.22*	56.4 ± 10.7	63.2 ± 10.4*
Fry and Kraemer, 1991	I	4.88 ± 0.27#		72.6 ± 9.3^	
	II	4.92 ± 0.26		69.3 ± 8.5	
	III	4.96 ± 0.27		67.4 ± 8.8	
Schmidt, 1999	III	–	–	56.0 ± 6.7	63.0 ± 7.1*
Garstecki et al., 2004	I	4.74 ± 0.30*		80.1 ± 10.2*	
	II	4.88 ± 0.30		70.1 ± 12.1	

Notes: * = significantly different; # = significantly different than Division III only; ^ = significantly different than Division II and Division III. All data are reported as mean ± SD, except for Fry and Kraemer, 1991 who reported mean only. One result indicates linemen and skill position players were combined.

TABLE 4.3 Strength Comparisons Between Starters and Nonstarters in College Football Players: Position Comparisons

NCAA Division	1RM Bench Press (kg)											
	Offensive Linemen		Defensive Linemen		Linebacker		Offensive Backs		Wide Receivers		Defensive Backs	
	S	NS	S	NS	S	NS	S	NS	S	NS	S	NS
I	165.0*	149.4	172.5*	151.6	157.1*	152.7	144.5*	138.5	130.2	121.2	134.7	131.0
II	163.2*	140.3	163.0*	135.9	152.0	137.7	137.1*	126.6	123.5	112.5	128.4	121.6
III	138.7	128.3	134.2	121.2	163.3	121.5	121.6	111.4	150.3^	127.0	139.8#	134.2
	1RM Squat (kg)											
I	212.2	209.5	231.5*	201.9	215.0	203.7	189.3	166.9	163.2	173.3	185.0	176.8
II	205.6	206.9	207.3	188.2	188.4	180.0	187.7	170.8	173.0	159.2	188.7	154.4
III	177.3	195.5	163.2	193.4	166.6	203.6	189.5	166.8	165.4	167.0	166.0	165.7
	1RM Power Clean (kg)											
I	133.5*	127.2	135.4	124.4	138.6*^	134.9	119.8*	109.5	117.9	107.8	122.1	112.3
II	127.1*	126.6	133.3	112.4	124.2	114.7	117.4	107.1	116.0	99.6	116.1	101.5
III	118.3	112.8	127.4	119.1	121.9	112.6	103.9	97.0	116.5	100.4	123.7	100.2

Source: Data from Fry and Kraemer, 1991.

Notes: All data are reported as group means. * = significantly greater than Division III; ^ = significantly greater than Division II; # = significantly greater than Division I.

noted between starters and nonstarters in the bench press exercise in offensive and defensive linemen, linebackers, running backs, and defensive backs. Significant differences between starters and nonstarters in the squat exercise were seen in running backs only, while significant differences in the power clean were noted between starters and nonstarters in defensive linemen, linebackers, running backs, wide receivers, and defensive backs. Starters were significantly faster than nonstarters for defensive linemen, linebackers, defensive backs, and wide receivers. Vertical jump height was significantly greater for starters than nonstarters in all positions except running backs. Greater strength and power in starters compared to nonstarters have also been demonstrated in other studies (Barker et al., 1993; Black and Roundy, 1994).

TABLE 4.4 Speed and Vertical Jump Comparisons Between Starters and Nonstarters in College Football: Position Comparisons

NCAA Division	40-yard Sprint (s)											
	Offensive Linemen		Defensive Linemen		Linebackers		Offensive Backs		Wide Receivers		Defensive Backs	
	S	NS	S	NS	S	NS	S	NS	S	NS	S	NS
I	5.09	5.16	4.88	5.02	4.74	4.91	4.73*	4.79	4.64	4.81	4.61	4.76
II	5.23	5.19	4.94	5.11	4.81	4.93	4.78*	4.82	4.65	4.85	4.61	4.82
III	5.22	5.26	4.96	5.20	4.80	4.99	4.85	4.93	4.72	4.86	4.67	4.81
	Vertical Jump (cm)											
I	69.5*^	63.3	72.3	56.9	74.5*	72.0	76.5*	73.7	77.1	73.2	82.5	72.7
II	64.0	61.1	71.9	64.7	71.7	68.1	72.3*	69.3	75.0	69.0	79.5	69.5
III	62.5	56.6	70.5	63.3	71.5	63.0	67.1	65.0	74.2	69.5	77.6	66.5

Source: Data from Fry and Kraemer, 1991.

Notes: All data are reported as group means. * = significantly better than Division III; ^ = significantly better than Division II.

In 1994, Black and Roundy published combined data from 11 NCAA Division I football programs collected between 1987 and 1991. They compared 16 positions and reported that one-repetition maximum (1RM) in the squat exercise was significantly different between starters and nonstarters for outside linebackers, cornerbacks, guards, tight ends, wide receivers, and running backs. Starters were also stronger than nonstarters in the 1RM bench press for defensive tackles, inside linebackers, cornerbacks, free safeties, all offensive linemen (centers, guards, and tackles), tight ends, quarterbacks, and fullbacks. Vertical jump height was different between starters and nonstarters for outside linebackers, cornerbacks, and wide receivers, while faster times in the 40-yard sprint were reported in starting defensive tackles, outside linebackers, cornerbacks, centers, guards, wide receivers, and quarterbacks compared to nonstarters in these positions. Cornerbacks were the only position that each of the performance variables was able to discriminate between starters and nonstarters. Interestingly, differentiation between starters and nonstarters was observed in three of the four performance measures among guards, outside linebackers, and wide receivers. Lower body strength, power, and speed appeared to differentiate between starters and nonstarters for both outside linebackers and wide receivers, while both upper and lower body strength, as well as speed, appeared to be able to differentiate playing ability in guards. These results are consistent with the requirements of each of these respective positions. Hoffman and Hamilton (2002) compared force outputs in offensive and defensive linemen in a wall-mounted sled. They reported that starters had a significantly greater force output than nonstarters in a sport-specific movement. This is the only study known that compared force outputs to playing time using a sport-specific movement.

As college football teams began to emphasize the strength and conditioning program, significant improvements were noted in athletic performance. The trend toward these improvements can be seen in Tables 4.1 and 4.2. Secora and colleagues (2004) compared performance changes in NCAA Division I football players from data published in 1990 (Berg et al., 1990). The investigators of the 1990 study sent surveys to the strength and conditioning coach or head football coach of 65 NCAA Division I universities, including all of the top final 20 ranked teams for 1987. Teams were requested to send the performance testing data of their 22 starters on the offensive and defensive teams. A total of 40 universities participated in the survey, including 17 of the teams that were ranked in the final top 20 poll. The focus of the study was not to compare starters and nonstarters, but to compare teams and conferences around the country and to determine how physical ability (e.g., speed, strength, and power) impacted football playing performance. The results of the Berg et al. (1990) study demonstrated that significant differences (p < 0.01) were noted between ranked and unranked teams in three of the ten variables measured: vertical jump height, vertical jump power, and bench press strength. These differences ranged from 4.1% to 5.2%. Vertical jump power was the only variable that was significantly correlated (r = −0.52, p < 0.05) to the final top 20 rankings. This was the first study to show a direct

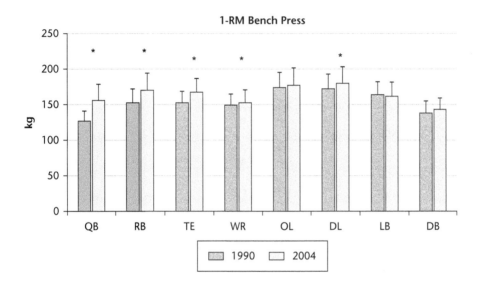

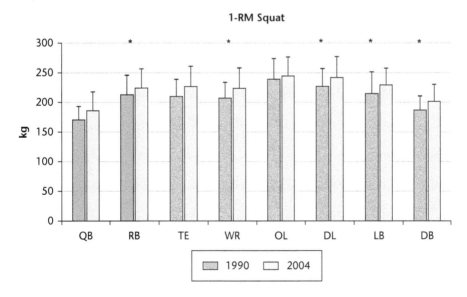

FIGURE 4.1   1990–2004 Comparisons in 1RM Bench Press (a), 1RM Squat (b), Vertical Jump Height (c), and 40-yard (36.6 m) Sprint Times (d). ★ = significant difference between years. All data are reported as mean ± SD.

Source: Data from Berg et al. (1990) and Secora et al. (2004).

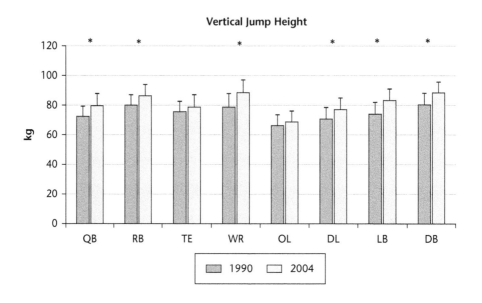

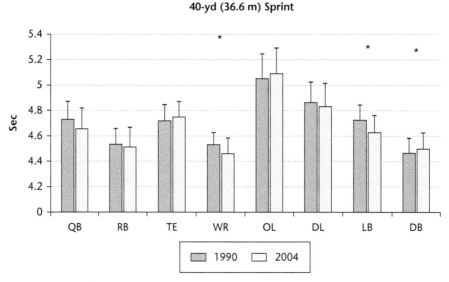

FIGURE 4.1 (Continued)

association between physical performance and football playing ability. Subsequent research has supported these results. A study by Sawyer and colleagues (2002) examined 40 NCAA Division I football players. All players were ranked by their football playing ability by their coaches, which was then compared to performance measures. Only vertical jump performance was significantly correlated to players ranking on both offense ($r = -0.50$, $p = 0.02$) and defense ($r = -0.64$, $p = 0.003$). Strength measures (1RM bench press and power clean) were significantly correlated to football playing ability for defensive players only ($r = -0.48$, $p = 0.03$, and $r = -0.58$, $p = 0.009$, respectively). Speed was significantly correlated (r's ranging from 0.58 to 0.63, $p < 0.05$) to football playing ability in skill position players only (wide receivers, defensive backs, linebackers, tight ends, and running backs).

Since the Berg et al. study (1990), the importance placed on the strength and conditioning programs in college football began to blossom. A greater commitment to the strength and conditioning program led to significant performance gains. Figure 4.1 provides a positional comparison between Berg et al. (1990) and Secora et al. (2004) in strength (1RM bench press and squat), vertical jump height, and speed, respectively. In the 14–15 years between studies, the greatest improvements were seen in the power measure (vertical jump height). Six of the eight positions measured (quarterbacks, running backs, wide receivers, defensive linemen, linebackers, and defensive backs) experienced significant improvements in power. This was consistent with the importance that power was reported to have on football playing ability (Berg et al., 1990; Sawyer et al., 2002). Only offensive linemen and tight ends did not improve. The position group that was shown to improve in all facets of physical ability during that ~15-year span were the wide receivers. Sprint speed was only improved in wide receivers and linebackers highlighting how difficult speed improvement is (see Chapter 3), and the important role that genetics plays in speed expression.

The effort to improve the physical conditioning of football players led to greater focus on the development of training facilities within NCAA Division I universities around the United States. Further increases in size, staffing, and budget were highlighted in a paper published by Judge and colleagues (2014). A total of 285 requests to participate in this survey were submitted to Division I strength coaches around the country. A total of 110 coaches responded to this request. The average size of the strength and conditioning facility was reported to be 7,017 square feet (652 m²). However, this included schools that had and didn't have football programs. Schools that had football programs, the average size of the facility was 9,949 square feet (924 m²). It is also important to note that not all facilities are dedicated to the football team, but often all athletic teams have access to the strength and conditioning facility. For football playing schools, strength and conditioning programs have about three facilities for use by their athletic teams. In these situations, a single strength and conditioning facility may be dedicated to the football program. These facilities had on average four full-time strength coaches, two part-time coaches, and three graduate assistants. Large strength and conditioning programs have approximately nine staff members per facility.

Despite the increase in facilities and staff of strength and conditioning programs in college football, there has been no further update regarding normative values of college football players since 2004. There have been a number of publications using college football players as subjects, examining different training programs, the impact of various supplements, or nutritional practices, but none of these investigations have provided any comparison data between starters and nonstarters or compared conferences or teams.

Performance Comparisons in Professional Football Players

Our understanding of performance capacity in NFL players is very limited. Although data are limited in these athletes, one of the first studies to examine football players was conducted on NFL players (Wilmore and Haskell, 1972). They examined 44 players who played for several teams in the NFL, including 9 "All-Pro" players. Data collection occurred between 1969 and 1972. They examined body composition and aerobic capacity of these players. The body composition data will be discussed in a later section of this chapter. The aerobic capacity of these players averaged 50.1 ml·kg·min^{-1} with a range between 40.1 and 60.0 ml·kg·min^{-1}. Positional comparisons showed that defensive linemen had the lowest aerobic capacity (43.5 ml·kg·min^{-1}), while defensive backs had the highest aerobic capacity (54.5 ml·kg·min^{-1}). The data collected by the investigators were consistent with the focus of athlete assessment during that time period. Most if not all exercise scientists during that generation focused on aerobic capacity as a gold standard measurement of any athlete, regardless of whether that measure had any association with specific athletic performance. A subsequent study examined physical performance measures in 167 professional players over a four-year period (1979–1982) (Shields et al., 1984). Strength was assessed using isokinetic and isometric measurements, while cardiovascular fitness was assessed by a run to exhaustion on a treadmill. In addition, body composition, flexibility, and reaction tests were also employed. Players were classified as rookies who were all nonstarters, veterans who were nonstarters, and finally veterans who were starters. No differences were noted in any of the strength or other performance measures between starters and nonstarters. However, starters (47.2 ± 5.1 ml·kg·min^{-1}) had a significantly higher aerobic capacity than nonstarters (44.2 ± 4.1 to 46.8 ± 6.1 ml·kg·min^{-1} in rookies and nonstarting veterans, respectively). In addition, the starters were also older than nonstarters. Results were somewhat surprising, but it should be acknowledged that the strength and conditioning profession was in its infancy during those years, and if those players were resistance training, it was likely not on the equipment that they were assessed on. Further, during that era, many coaches were under the belief that aerobic capacity, even for strength/power athletes, had important performance-related benefits. It took years to overcome and convince coaches of this specific training myth.

In the 1980s, many professional football teams required their players to perform a 1.5-mile run as part of their conditioning assessments. Offensive linemen were required to finish in 12 min or less; if not, they were forced to run again the next day or until they passed. Although it was not understood during that time period, it was clearly a violation of the specificity principle. However, it was not the only anaerobic sport that was making that mistake. Future Hall-of-Fame basketball coach Jim Calhoun at the University of Connecticut was a big believer in his players performing a 2-mile run prior to each season. As the strength coach, he provided me the opportunity to train the players in the manner I deemed best, with no interference, but he insisted that this endurance test be performed. No discussion was going to convince him otherwise. After four years of testing (the 2-mile run and more appropriate strength, speed, agility, and power assessment), there were sufficient data to examine the worthiness of endurance testing in anaerobic athletes. The relationship of all performance tests performed, including the 2-mile run, to playing time was examined. Endurance performance actually was shown to be significantly related to playing time, albeit a negative relationship (Hoffman et al., 1996). Those players who had the highest aerobic capacity played the least. The players with the lowest aerobic capacity but with great lower body strength, power, and speed went on to play the more significant minutes. To provide some perspective to this, six of the players who played on those teams at UCONN during the 1988–1992 seasons became #1 draft picks in the NBA.

It was many years before any additional performance measures were published in NFL players. Pryor and colleagues (2014) examined players from the Super Bowl XLVI winning New York Giants. The investigation focused primarily on body composition measures, but the investigators also reported on maximal strength, which was estimated from the players training logbooks taken from the final week of the strength phase of the athlete's periodized training program. This was the first study to provide strength data, albeit predicted, on NFL players from a single team. The investigators provided positional comparisons. As might be expected, offensive and defensive linemen appeared to be the strongest players in the 1RM bench press and squat exercises. Significant differences were also noted in the 1RM bench press between positions; wide receivers were significantly weaker than offensive and defensive linemen and linebackers; tight ends were significantly weaker than offensive linemen, and defensive backs were significantly weaker than all linemen, linebackers, and running backs. The only significant difference noted in the 1RM squat exercise was between offensive linemen and wide receivers. No significant positional differences were noted in the 1RM power clean. Whether strength, speed, agility, or power measures can differentiate between starters and nonstarters at the professional level is still not well-understood. Obviously, these athletes are strong, fast, and powerful. Whether a NFL athlete who can squat

275 kg is a better player than one playing the same position and can squat 250 kg is difficult to ascertain, and it is debatable. With all things considered – rate of force development, technique, nutrition, toughness, etc., there are a host of potential variables that contribute to success at this level of competition. If everything was equal, except for strength, then it would likely have a great impact.

Performance differences between positions do appear to be specific to the needs of each position. Linemen are the biggest players and they are also the strongest. Their position requires them to engage their opponent on every play and assist or deny (depending on which side of the ball) the skill position players from executing their job. Wide receivers and defensive backs rely on their speed and agility to create or close windows of opportunity. Strength is not their primary weapon, but being strong does provide certain positional advantages. For instance, strong receivers would be more successful in blocking or releasing off the line of scrimmage as they are being "pressed" by the defensive back. Greater strength for a defensive back would assist in overpowering blockers, especially wide receivers, but also provide an advantage in "press" coverage, in which they are trying to jam the wide receiver at the line of scrimmage. Running backs and linebackers have some similarity within their strength and speed characteristics. Their responsibilities generally parallel each other.

Power, Speed, and Agility Comparisons in High School Football Players

The number of studies examining normative data in high school football players is much fewer than that seen at the collegiate level. This is most likely related to the lack of sport scientists in high schools and the accessibility to those athletes. There have been two major publications

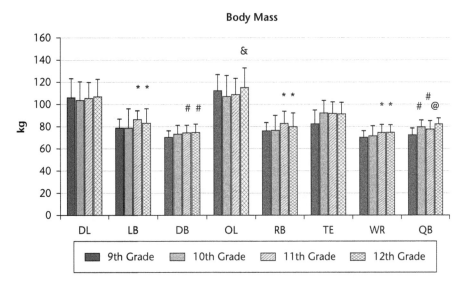

FIGURE 4.2 Grade Comparisons of High School Football Players in Body Mass (a), 40-yard (36.6 m) Sprint Times (b), Pro-Agility Time (c), Vertical Jump Height (d), and Vertical Jump Power (e). ★ = significantly different from 9th and 10th grades; # = significantly different from 9th grade only; ^ = significantly different from 10th grade only; & = significantly different from 11th grade only; @ = significantly different from 9th and 11th grades; $ = significantly different from 10th and 11th grades. All data are reported as mean ± SD.

Source: Data from Dupler et al., 2010.

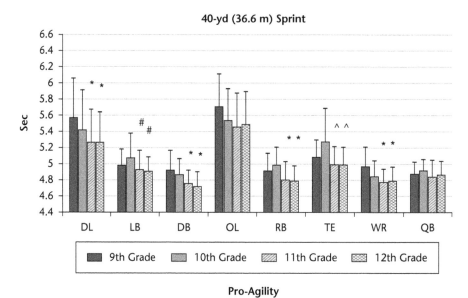

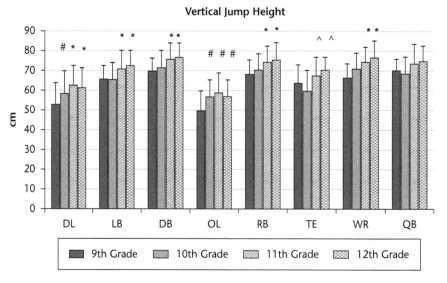

FIGURE 4.2 (Continued)

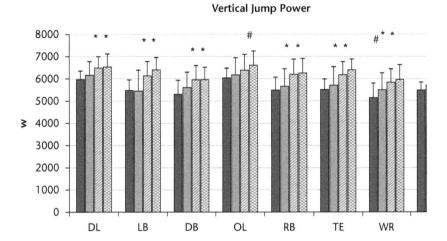

FIGURE 4.2 (Continued)

that have provided normative data on large groups of high school football players. However, these studies focused on the speed and agility of the athletes and not on strength measures. The first study was published by Terry Dupler and colleagues (2010) who examined power (vertical jump height), speed (40-yard sprint times), and agility (pro-agility) in 2,327 high school players participating in the Texas high school combine. The data from this study appear in Figure 4.2. The results appeared to differentiate underclassmen (9th and 10th grades) and upperclassmen (11th and 12th grades). This supports the concept of having younger players participate in junior varsity football and upperclassmen play varsity. Body mass gains in high school football players during their four-years of play ranged from 0.8 kg in defensive linemen to 10.1 kg in quarterbacks. The large gain in body mass among quarterbacks may have contributed to the lack of change in 40-yard sprint speed during their high school careers. Regardless, there appeared to be only limited improvements in any of the speed or agility measures between the ninth and tenth grades. Although improvements were seen in these variables starting in the 11th grade, only tight ends experienced further improvements in agility performance between 11th and 12th grades. Similar to what was observed in college athletes, improvements in speed and agility can occur, but these changes do appear to plateau during the high school players junior year. In examining raw scores, the change in 40-yard sprint times ranged from −0.01 s (quarterbacks) to −0.30 s (defensive linemen) during the four-year high school career. These results were similar to a more recent examination of changes in speed in high school football players tested at various combines around the United States (Leutzinger et al., 2018). In that study, changes in speed between 9th and 11th graders ranged from −0.11 s in tight ends to −0.26 s in defensive linemen. Interestingly, the greatest improvements were noted in the slowest positions – both offensive and defensive lines, for both studies. Dupler and colleagues (2010) reported that all positions improved vertical jump and vertical jump power during the four years of high school play. However, no improvements were noted between the 11th and 12th grade in any of the power measures.

The study by Leutzinger and colleagues (2018) examined 7,160 high school football players participating in 12 different high school American football recruiting combines throughout the United States. Changes in body mass in this cross-sectional study ranged from 6 kg (tight ends and wide receivers) to 12 kg in defensive ends. Significant improvements were also noted in both vertical jump height (ranging from +2.7 cm in defensive ends to +8.0 cm in defensive backs) and pro-agility time (ranging from −0.09 s in defensive tackles to −0.17 s in both linebackers and offensive linemen) in all high school players.

Body Composition of Football Players

The body composition and body mass of college and professional football players can be seen in Table 4.5. One of the first studies reporting on body composition of football players examined 44 NFL players (Wilmore and Haskell, 1972). The body fat percentage of the linemen, which was assessed using hydrostatic weighing, was less than 20%. This was remarkably low in comparison to subsequent measures, but one needs to acknowledge that these players were likely not participating in any strength program. A subsequent study on 36 players from the Atlantic Falcons of the NFL used both hydrostatic weighing and skinfold measures to assess body composition (Snow et al., 1998). In the 26 years between these NFL studies, the weight gain between positions ranged from 3.7 kg in running backs to 2.5 kg in offensive linemen. These changes likely reflect the greater importance placed in the strength and conditioning programs of both collegiate and professional football teams. The latter study also reported body composition values from both hydrostatic weighing and skinfold measures. No differences were noted for any position except for offensive linemen. The skinfold measures appeared to underestimate the body fat percentage of these athletes. Although hydrostatic weighing had been considered the "gold" standard for body composition analysis at that time, there were issues raised with the body density equation. A study on Canadian professional football players actually reported negative values in some of their leaner athletes (both Caucasian and African American) (Adams et al., 1981). It was suggested that the bone density equations were likely not race appropriate or specific for this population group.

Investigations examining body composition in NCAA football players have also been published. Smith and Mansfield (1984) investigated 68 members of the University of Alabama's football team during the 1980–1981 season. They used several different methods to analyze body fat and suggested that most models overestimated body density in players with actually low body density, and underestimated body density when body density was actually high. In a study conducted 20 years later, 69 NCAA Division I football players from Michigan State University were examined by investigators using several different skinfold formulas, as well as hydrostatic weighing (Noel et al., 2003). More than half of the players tested decided not to participate in the hydrostatic weighing, thus those results are not reported. Noel and colleagues (2003) reported that although college football players were getting bigger (i.e., heavier), their percent body fat was also increasing. The concern was raised regarding the potential health effects associated with greater body fat in these players. However, the impact of body composition on football performance was not considered, nor had it in any previous study. Stuempfle and colleagues (2003) examining 77 NCAA Division III college football players from Gettysburg College compared body composition results between starters and nonstarters, as well as examined the relationship between body composition (measured hydrostatically) and commonly used tests of performance, including speed, agility, power, and strength. No difference was seen in body fat composition between starters and nonstarters, and no relationship was noted between body fat composition and strength. Body fat percentage, however, was significantly correlated with 40-yard sprint

TABLE 4.5 Anthropometric Comparisons Between Positions in Football (Body Fat%/Body Mass)

Reference	Level of Play	Method of Assessment	Offensive Linemen	Offensive Backs	Wide Receivers	Tight Ends	Quarterbacks	Defensive Linemen	Linebackers	Defensive Backs
Wilmore and Haskell, 1972	NFL	Hydrostatic weighing	15.5%[1] 113.2 kg	8.3%[2] 91.8 kg	[2]	[1]	–	18.7% 120.6 kg	18.5% 107.6 kg	7.7% 85.0 kg
Smith and Mansfield, 1984	NCAA Division I	Skinfold	12.8% 98.5 kg	7.8% 89.1 kg	–	–	10.9% 84.5 kg	13.9% 111.3 kg	11.5% 94.6 kg	7.3% 83.2 kg
Snow et al., 1998	NFL	Hydrostatic weighing and skinfold	21.7 ± 4.2% 24.7 ± 4.7% 135.7 ± 13.4 kg	10.7 ± 4.7% 12.6 ± 4.8% 95.5 ± 17.8 kg	–	–	–	20.8 ± 4.8% 20.3 ± 2.9% 126.8 ± 8.7 kg	16.0 ± 2.2% 15.3 ± 2.6% 113.1 ± 8.0 kg	9.7 ± 1.7% 10.7 ± 1.4% 93.7 ± 5.6 kg
Noel et al., 2003	NCAA Division I	Skinfold	21.9 ± 2.0%[1] 122.4 ± 4.7 kg	9.0 ± 2.1%[2] 86.6 ± 2.9 kg	[2]	[1]	11.8 ± 3.1% 84.8 ± 1.8 kg	20.9 ± 3.5% 110.5 ± 5.4 kg	13.9 ± 4.4% 104.1 ± 4.7 kg	9.0 ± 1.2% 86.9 ± 1.3 kg
Stuempfle et al., 2003	NCAA Division III	Hydrostatic weighing	21.9 ± 4.5% 101.0 ± 9.2 kg	13.8 ± 3.3 79.6 ± 6.0	–	–	–	21.5 ± 4.5 96.6 ± 7.9 kg	–	15.2 ± 4.6% 85.7 ± 6.5 kg
Kraemer et al., 2005	NFL	Plethysmography	25.1 ± 2.5% 140.0 ± 7.5 kg	7.3 ± 7.3% 96.5 ± 8.1 kg	8.1 ± 2.8% 85.6 ± 6.5 kg	15.1 ± 5.4% 115.6 ± 7.2 kg	14.6 ± 9.3% 104.2 ± 2.6 kg	18.5 ± 3.8% 126.8 ± 2.4 kg	15.7 ± 2.8% 107.8 ± 2.9 kg	6.3 ± 2.8% 87.1 ± 5.6 kg
Dengel et al., 2014	NFL	DEXA	28.8 ± 3.7% 140.9 ± 6.1 kg	16.0 ± 4.0% 105.4 ± 8.5 kg	12.5 ± 3.1% 94.0 ± 6.0 kg	16.8 ± 3.8% 113.9 ± 4.2 kg	19.6 ± 4.6% 103.6 ± 13.9 kg	25.2 ± 7.6% 132.9 ± 14.7 kg	17.0 ± 3.2% 109.9 ± 4.3 kg	12.1 ± 3.3% 90.8 ± 6.1 kg
Melvin et al., 2014	NCAA Div. I	DEXA	24.4 ± 2.2% 136.5 ± 11.0 kg	13.9 ± 2.0% 94.4 ± 10.2 kg	14.4 ± 2.2% 88.0 ± 6.6 kg	17.9 ± 2.8% 109.7 ± 6.6 kg	18.1 ± 2.1% 96.9 ± 2.1 kg	22.3 ± 2.3% 132.2 ± 9.4 kg	17.0 ± 2.9% 103.5 ± 3.9 kg	14.0 ± 2.2% 89.4 ± 6.3 kg
Pryor et al., 2014	NFL	Skinfold	21.9 ± 4.2% 144.0 ± 5.0 kg	14.1 ± 3.5% 110.5 ± 12.8 kg	5.2 ± 1.7% 86.4 ± 3.6 kg	18.7 ± 11.4% 123.3 ± 4.6 kg	13.3 ± 1.4% 100.9 ± 0.0 kg	19.4 ± 4.1% 134.7 ± 12.3 kg	11.7 ± 2.8% 108.1 ± 3.0 kg	10.2 ± 3.4% 90.0 ± 8.7 kg
Bosch et al., 2019	NCAA Div. I	DEXA	30.8 ± 4.2% 135.5 ± 11.8 kg	15.3 ± 3.9% 95.1 ± 9.6 kg	14.1 ± 3.6% 87.2 ± 8.8 kg	19.8 ± 3.9% 107.4 ± 9.6 kg	17.2 ± 4.2% 93.9 ± 8.2 kg	23.5 ± 7.0% 120.4 ± 14.2 kg	18.8 ± 4.9% 102.0 ± 6.6 kg	13.3 ± 3.2% 87.8 ± 6.5 kg

Notes: [1], [2] = Reported as one group; DEXA = dual-energy X-ray absorptiometry.

time (r = 0.70) and pro-agility (r = 0.52) and vertical jump (r = −0.59). However, partialing out body mass resulted in a reduction in these relationships (r = 0.47, 0.30, and −0.48 in the 40-yard sprint, pro-agility, and vertical jump tests). Regardless, body composition appeared to explain between 9% and 23% of the shared variance in these performance measures. Interestingly, a subsequent study in NCAA Division I athletes also reported no significant difference in body composition between starters (18.2 ± 4.3%) and nonstarters (17.7 ± 4.8%) (Melvin et al., 2014).

In 2005, another study examining the body composition of an NFL team (Indianapolis Colts) was published (Kraemer et al., 2005). Using plethysmography measurements, the entire Colts football team was assessed during summer training, prior to the start of the regular season (see Table 4.5). In comparison to the first publication in NFL players, in the 33 years between these papers the offensive linemen gained ~27 kg, defensive linemen gained ~6.8 kg, while backs increased approximately 5 kg of body mass. Although difficult to compare different body composition modalities, offensive linemen increased their body fat percentage by ~10%, running backs decreased their body fat percentage, and defensive linemen, despite the gain in body mass, did not change body fat percentage. Many of these changes were reflected in the study of the Atlanta Falcons seven years earlier (Snow et al., 1998). Some of the other positions such as linebackers actually maintained their body mass but lowered body fat. This was suggested to be related to the different styles of play (e.g., greater movement needs), conditioning programs, and nutritional interventions (Kraemer et al., 2005). A subsequent study of NFL players was conducted on the Green Bay Packers from 2006 to 2011 (Dengel et al., 2014). A total of 411 players (aged 20–38 years), who were active players on the roster, free agents, or prospective draft choices, were examined. Players were measured just before the NFL draft or before the start of the summer training camp using dual-energy X-ray absorptiometry (DEXA). The approximate ten-year difference between this study and that published by Kraemer et al. (2005) revealed that offensive linemen had a similar body mass, but defensive linemen were approximately 6 kg heavier (see Table 4.5). Increases in body mass were also noted in running backs (~9 kg) and wide receivers (~8.4 kg). Because of the difference in methodology used to assess body composition, it is difficult to make these comparisons. However, the benefit of using DEXA is that it can provide a measure of bone density, bone mineral content, and segmental measures of body composition.

The amount of lean mass in the upper and lower bodies of both offensive and defensive linemen appeared to be similar (Dengel et al., 2014). This is thought to be important as these positions are suggested to have a similar role as an anchor (Kraemer et al., 2005). These players do not want to give ground. Thus, a reduced upper body to lower body ratio, in regards to lean body mass, would provide a better anchor than a player who is top heavy (e.g., a high upper body to lower body ratio).

Body composition profiles of NFL players, as well as all football players, are quite interesting. In general, these are very big men who are in very good physical condition. However, if procedures used to assess obesity are applied to this subject population (e.g., body mass index), most players would be considered to be obese. The body composition values for most positions are near normal values, except for linemen. Although these players are in good physical condition, their body fat percentage has generated concern for their long-term health (Snow et al., 1998; Bosch et al., 2014). Body fat percentages greater than 25% in both offensive and defensive linemen are indicative of these players being overfat or obese. Bosch and colleagues (2014) reported that visceral adipose tissue was significantly greater in the linemen compared to all other position groups. Greater body fat likely serves to protect internal organs and bone structures for these specific positions that are involved in contact with every play. However, the accumulation of visceral adipose tissue does increase cardiovascular health risks in these athletes. This potential risk, especially during the players' retirement, will be discussed in greater detail in Chapter 7.

Pryor and colleagues (2014) published anthropometric data from returning players of the Super Bowl XLVI winning New York Giants team at the beginning of the 2012 off-season training. Body composition was assessed using skinfold measurements. Although a small sample size was examined, a trend toward a reduction in body fat was noted (except in tight ends and running backs) and a lower or similar body mass (with the exception of tight ends and defensive linemen) was noted in comparison to previous studies examining NFL players (Kraemer et al., 2005; Snow et al., 1998).

In 2019, Bosch and colleagues pooled anthropometric data from several NCAA Division I football programs (Texas Christian University, University of Texas at Austin, University of Kansas, and University of Minnesota). The data of 467 athletes who were tested in multiple years between 2011 and 2016 were analyzed. All athletes were assessed with DEXA scans, and all scans were conducted during preseason training (June–July). In comparison to previous data using similar assessment tools (Melvin et al., 2014), offensive linemen, running backs, and tight ends increased body fat % (>3.0%), while no changes (<1.0%) were noted for the other positions. Interestingly, increases in body fat were not accompanied by any change in body mass, indicating that players in these positions were fatter. However, this does not suggest that the greater body fat was associated with poor football playing performance. In fact, as discussed earlier in the chapter, body composition is not associated with football playing performance. It is possible that changes in body fat percentage may explain changes in performance. For instance, a gain in body fat may explain why a player was slower or less agile, and a decrease in body fat may provide a partial explanation of why performance improved.

Positional comparisons of total bone mineral density (BMD) in NCAA Division I college football players can be observed in Figure 4.3. The positions with the greatest total BMD were, as expected, the linemen, while the lowest total BMD was observed in the skill position players (Bosch et al., 2019). Total BMD ranged from 1.65 g·cm² in defensive linemen to 1.51 g·cm² in wide receivers. The z-score for these athletes ranged from 2.1 (wide receivers) to 3.4 in offensive

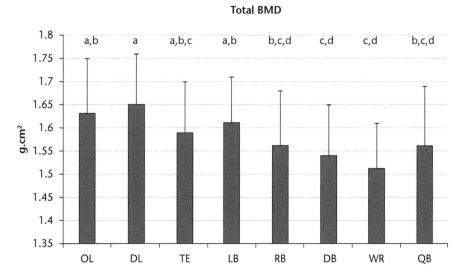

FIGURE 4.3   Total Bone Mineral Density (BMD) in NCAA Division I College Football Players. If position doesn't share a letter, it is significantly different. All data are reported as mean ± SD.

Source: Data from Bosch et al., 2019.

linemen. These results were similar to that reported in NFL players (Dengel et al., 2014). Dengel et al. (2014) reported on bone mineral content and bone density in the spine. These measures were highest among the linemen and tight ends. Bone mineral content ranged from 5.1 ± 0.4 kg in offensive linemen to 4.2 ± 0.3 kg in defensive backs (kickers were slightly lower), while bone density in the spine ranged from 1.59 g·cm^2 in offensive linemen to 1.45 ± 0.13 g·cm^2 in quarterbacks (although kickers were also slightly lower).

Predictive Ability of the National Football League Combine

The NFL combine has become a television extravaganza that is broadcast live for four days every February. The NFL invites approximately 330–340 of the top college football players who are draft-eligible to their combine. During the combine, each player is asked to complete an intelligence and problem-solving test (e.g., Wonderlic test) and a number of physical performance measures, including the anthropometric measures, speed (40-yard sprint), agility (pro-agility, 3-cone drill), power (vertical jump, broad jump), and strength [maximum number of repetitions with 225 lb (100 kg) in the bench press]. The NFL combine started in 1982. In the nearly 40 years that the combine has been operating, several investigations have been published examining whether it accomplishes what it purports to do; select the best players who will be successful in the NFL.

Each NFL team has an elaborate scouting system that covers the entire country scouting college football games looking to identify talent. The scouts focus is on the football playing traits of the player. Does he maintain effort throughout each play – the term does he have a "high motor" is often used, or does he take plays off? How is his technique? What happens when he is challenged? Does he play better or worse against good competition? All of these subjective or qualitative measures go into the scouting report. However, the quantitative analysis plays an important role as well. The players' height, size, limb length, strength, speed, power, and quickness – are they competitive for a NFL player. These quantitative assessments provide another measure for consideration by the team's general manager, whose job is dependent upon the success of his draft picks. This understanding has resulted in a cottage industry of elite training facilities that cater to players preparing for the NFL combine. The importance of performing well on these tests is simply a financial one. The higher the player is drafted, the more money he will make. There is little to no negotiation room for rookie contracts. They are all for four years, and no renegotiation can occur until after year 3. This is according to the NFL players association bargaining agreement. Thus, where the player gets drafted will determine what his contract will be. The first pick of the 2020 draft is projected to earn $36,000,000 in his four-year contract with a $24.5 million signing bonus. The subsequent draft picks will get less. Table 4.6 provides the average projected salary per round for the 2020 draft (Spotrac, 2020).

TABLE 4.6 NFL Draft: Rookie Salaries Projected 2020

Round	Total Salary (Four Years)	Bonus
1	$17,844,465	$10,937,793
2	$6,346,930	$2,575,949
3	$3,999,269	$1,018,778
4	$3,283,954	$748,954
5	$2,857,228	$322,228
6	$2,713,977	$178,977
7	$2,630,036	$95,036

Source: Data from www.spotrac.com/nfl/draft/

The first paper published on the NFL combine was conducted with the data of 326 college players who were invited to the 2000 NFL combine (McGee and Burkett, 2003). The investigators used the performance measures collected during the combine and created a regression equation for each position on the players who were drafted to determine the predictability of these equations. The results of this investigation indicated that the regression equations were able to predict the draft round of prospective NFL quarterbacks with a high degree of success: $r^2 = 0.84$. The greatest predictor for the quarterbacks was the 3-cone drill. This value indicates that performance in the 3-cone drill was able to explain 84% of the variance of the draft selection. However, this measure does very little to describe the most important needs of a quarterback such as arm strength, accuracy, decision-making ability, and leadership. This suggests that there is likely a degree of overlap between performance in the 3-cone drill and other factors that were not inputted into the equation. Regression equations for offensive and defensive linemen were $r^2 = 0.70$ and $r^2 = 0.59$, respectively. Performance measures that were the best predictors for success for these athletes were height, weight, bench press, 3-cone drill, and the broad jump. The regression equation had limited success ($r^2 = 0.22$) in predicting draft order for linebackers. However, it had great success for running backs, wide receivers, and defensive backs ($r^2 = 1.0$ for all positions) in determining draft round. The importance of speed and agility for these positions put large emphasis on these tests at the combine. These results were supported by a subsequent study that compared players who participated in the 2004 and 2005 combines, and either were or were not drafted (Sierer et al., 2008). Players who were drafted performed significantly better in the combine tests than those players who were not drafted. Specifically, skill position players who were drafted performed significantly better in the 40-yard sprint, vertical jump, pro-agility, and 3-cone drills than undrafted skill players. Linemen who were drafted performed significantly better in the bench press, 40-yard sprint, and the 3-cone drill than undrafted linemen.

In 2008, a study was published that examined the ability of the NFL combine to predict football playing performance in the NFL (Kuzmits and Adams, 2008). The investigators used the combine performance measures (10-, 20-, and 40-yard sprints, bench press, vertical jump, broad jump, 20- and 60-yard shuttles, 3-cone drill, and the Wonderlic test). The performance criteria used included draft order, three year totals of salary received, games played, and position-specific data. The data were aggregated for six years (1999–2004). The correlational analysis determined that the combine results provided no meaningful degree of predictive validity for NFL performance, except for the relationship between sprint times and running back success. Subsequent research, examining only running backs and wide receivers, also indicated that combine data had predictive ability for future play in the NFL for those positions (Teramoto et al., 2016). In their analysis, the investigators accounted for the number of games played, draft position, height, and body mass. They determined that 10-yard sprint time was the most important predictor of rushing yards per attempt in the running backs' first three years of their career, while vertical jump performance was found to be significantly associated with receiving yards per reception during the athletes' first three years of their career. Although these studies found some value in the predictability of combine data, most of the performance measures examined were found not to be very useful.

The validity of the NFL combine does appear to be limited. Much of this is likely related to lack of specificity of tests and a concern of potential injury preventing a more appropriate testing battery. For instance, the 225 lb (102 kg) bench press test for repetitions has absolutely no value as a strength measure. Once an athlete performs more than ten repetitions in the exercise, the validity to predict strength is lost (Mayhew et al., 1999). Further, there is no measure for lower body strength. Considering that strength is an important variable for football performance,

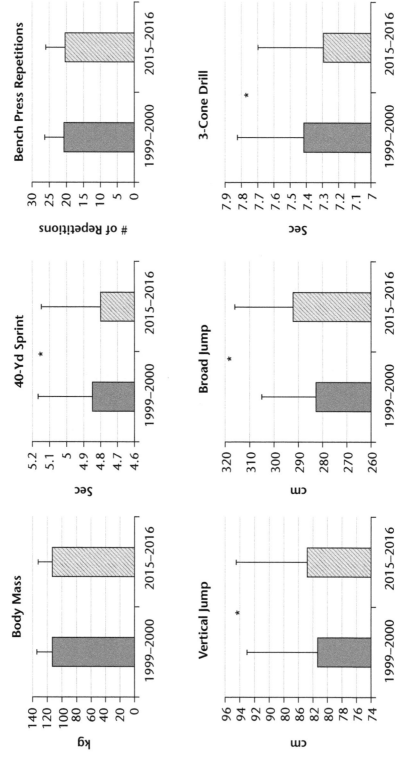

FIGURE 4.4 Comparison of NFL Combine Data from 1999–2000 to 2015–2016. ★ = significantly different. All data are reported as mean ± SD.

Source: Data from Fitzgerald and Jensen, 2020.

especially for linemen, it is surprising that no assessment of strength is performed at the NFL combine. To date, speed, vertical jump, and agility appear to be the most important performance variables being assessed at the combine.

There have been a few studies that have examined the change in performance data over time at the NFL combine (Fitzgerald and Jensen, 2020; Robbins et al., 2013). Robbins and colleagues (2013) compared data of a ten-year span (1999–2001 to 2008–2010). Their results indicated that all positions were faster in the 10-yard (9.1 m), 20-yard (18.2 m), and 40-yard (36.6 m) sprint, except for defensive tackles, fullbacks, and quarterbacks who remained the same in the 40-yard sprint only. No changes were noted in either the pro-agility or vertical jump height in any position. In addition, 9 of 13 football positions identified improved the number of repetitions in the bench press exercise. Whether this indicates the players were stronger is highly debatable, but it does indicate a greater attention in preparing for this assessment. Fitzgerald and Jensen (2020) compared the 1999–2000 combine data to the combine data of 2015–2016. A total of 1,263 football players were examined. The results of all positions combined can be observed in Figure 4.4. In the ~15 years separating the two data sets, significant improvements were observed in 40-yard sprint speed, 3-cone drill, vertical jump, and broad jump performance. No changes were noted in height, body mass, pro-agility time, and the number of repetitions performed in the bench press test. When performing position-specific comparisons (see Table 4.7), significant increases in body mass were noted in quarterbacks, wide receivers, and tight ends. Improved times were observed in the 40-yard sprint in running backs, wide receivers, defensive and offensive linemen, and defensive backs. No improvements were noted for the number of repetitions in the bench press and vertical jump performance. However, all positions significantly improved

TABLE 4.7 Fifteen-Year Performance Comparisons of Players Participating in the NFL Combine

Position	Year	Body Mass (kg)	40-yard Sprint (s)	Bench Press (reps)	Vertical Jump (cm)	Broad Jump (cm)	Pro Agility (s)	3-Cone Drill (s)
QB	1999–2,000	98.3 ± 5.6	4.91 ± 0.27	–	79.6 ± 8.1	273.7 ± 17.7	4.39 ± 0.17	7.37 ± 0.20
	2015–2,016	101.8 ± 5.8*	4.81 ± 0.16	–	80.7 ± 7.6	287.1 ± 16.9*	4.29 ± 0.16*	7.10 ± 0.19*
RB	1999–2,000	99.5 ± 4.9	4.74 ± 0.27	19.2 ± 3.8	87.1 ± 8.9	295.5 ± 15.9	4.23 ± 0.19	7.13 ± 0.30
	2015–2,016	99.8 ± 6.9	4.58 ± 0.12*	19.8 ± 4.7	88.0 ± 8.3	301.8 ± 14.3*	4.26 ± 0.13	7.10 ± 0.19
WR	1999–2,000	89.5 ± 6.9	4.75 ± 0.29	–	89.5 ± 6.2	297.4 ± 13.1	4.17 ± 0.13	7.15 ± 0.21
	2015–2,016	92.5 ± 6.4*	4.52 ± 0.10*	14.0 ± 3.6	89.5 ± 8.3	307.2 ± 14.7*	4.22 ± 0.13*	6.97 ± 0.20*
TE	1999–2,000	117.1 ±5.9	4.85 ± 0.23	20.3 ± 4.5	80.3 ± 7.6	281.9 ± 16.0	4.37 ± 0.19	7.36 ± 0.33
	2015–2,016	114.3 ± 4.0*	4.79 ± 0.12	19.3 ± 4.3	84.0 ± 7.0	293.4 ± 12.1*	4.39 ± 0.14	7.00 ± 0.09*
DL	1999–2,000	129.3 ± 8.5	4.90 ± 0.28	23.6 ± 5.9	78.0 ± 7.3	274.6 ± 16.0	4.48 ± 0.19	7.62 ± 0.33
	2015–2,016	130.0 ± 11.8	4.97 ± 0.20*	25.1 ± 4.7	80.0 ± 9.4	283.4 ± 19.9*	4.53 ± 0.22	7.50 ± 0.34*
OL	1999–2,000	142.7 ± 8.6	5.02 ± 0.34	24.1 ± 5.0	69.1 ± 6.8	253.5 ± 14.9	4.71 ± 0.19	7.92 ± 0.29
	2015–2,016	141.8 ± 6.6	5.26 ± 0.18*	24.7 ± 4.9	71.0 ± 8.6	260.4 ± 18.4*	4.73 ± 0.18	7.85 ± 0.32
LB	1999–2,000	110.1 ± 4.2	4.89 ± 0.34	19.9 ± 4.6	84.3 ± 6.4	289.8 ± 11.0	4.30 ± 0.12	7.38 ± 0.28
	2015–2,016	109.4 ± 4.6	4.81 ± 0.56	20.6 ± 3.7	84.4 ± 8.4	296.6 ± 16.2*	4.32 ± 0.16	7.16 ± 0.27*
DB	1999–2,000	88.7 ± 5.6	4.70 ± 0.29	15.3 ± 4.2	91.3 ± 5.5	302.7 ± 11.6	4.16 ± 0.15	7.07 ± 0.26
	2015–2,016	89.0 ± 5.0	4.53 ± 0.10*	15.5 ± 3.8	90.7 ± 6.9	309.1 ± 15.6*	4.17 ± 0.14	6.99 ± 0.17*

Source: Data from Fitzgerald and Jensen, 2020.

Notes: QB = quarterback; RB = running back; WR = wide receiver; TE = tight end; DL = defensive line; OL = offensive line; LB = linebacker; DB = defensive back; * = significantly different. All data are reported as mean ± SD.

broad jump performance. Only running backs were observed to improve pro-agility time, but wide receivers actually became significantly slower. Still, all positions improved the other agility measure (3-cone drill), except for running backs and offensive linemen.

The changes in performance for the 15-year study appear to reflect the importance that speed and agility have in the game. The 40-yard sprint test and vertical jump are the only measures that have been associated with greater football performance in running backs and wide receivers (Teramoto et al., 2016). However, this is likely a perception for all positions, and it is emphasized by many of the training facilities that have popped up all over the United States to prepare football players for the combine. The focus of the sports performance industry is preparing their clients for the NFL combine. Considering that the broad jump has little specificity to football performance, the significant improvements seen in all positions likely reflect the emphasis placed on that test in the athlete's preparation for the combine.

Summary

With the growth of the strength and conditioning profession, a tremendous emphasis in the past 40 years has been placed on improving the performance capabilities of competitive football players. This is reflected with the tremendous increases in strength and power at all levels of play. Interestingly, most of the research examining the relationship between specific performance variables and playing time occurred during the first 20 years of the profession. However, the academic study of strength and conditioning has appeared to become stagnant in the twenty-first century. There may be a number of reasons for this. Part of this may be related to competitive issues, the amount of money in the game, and coaches who may have less desire to share their data with colleagues. Further, the catastrophic injuries that have occurred in preseason football in the past 20 years have created a bit of mistrust and a "circle-the-wagon" atmosphere that has limited the collaborative potential of athletic programs with the academic exercise/sport science faculty.

The NFL combine has become more of a sideshow to hold the interest of football fans during the spring. The combine begins the countdown to the NFL draft and keeps the NFL relevant in the public eye. It has made football a 12-month sport. Scientifically speaking, the question of whether the NFL combine provides any meaningful data is questionable. The limited amount of research has not been favorable, but it does suggest that speed and vertical jump height are important for skill position players. It is likely that the strength data for the scouts is provided by the athletes' strength coaches from their respective universities and is not gathered at the combine. Risk for injury and the complexity for strength assessment of more than 300 athletes likely limit this from being a realistic measure to be done at the combine.

5

NUTRITION, HYDRATION, AND DIETARY SUPPLEMENTATION FOR THE AMERICAN FOOTBALL PLAYER

Introduction

The field of sport nutrition is even younger than the strength and conditioning profession. Although nutritionists have been around a long time, the idea of someone focusing on the diet of competitive athletes is something that has only gained traction in the last 20–25 years. This is likely related to the exploding nutritional supplement industry that required athletes and teams to provide some direction for their players. For many years, athletes were generally on their own or relied upon their coaches to provide advice. In the past 25 years, much knowledge has been gained. However, despite sport nutritionists working with nearly every professional football team and most NCAA Division I football programs, the number of research studies specifically conducted on American football pales in comparison to soccer, rugby, and most other sports. As support programs around each program grow, the science providing a level of efficacy and validity to specific dietary interventions is not keeping pace in football. Much of the knowledge that is gained is unfortunately extrapolated from other sports.

In this chapter, I will focus on reviewing basic sport nutrition, both macro- and micronutrient intakes, and how it can be applied to the football player. In addition, the importance of hydration will also be covered. How much do football players know about their nutrition is an interesting topic, which will also be discussed. Finally, the popular nutritional supplements specific to the football player will be reviewed.

Importance of Nutrition for Athletic Performance

I was the strength coach for the University of Connecticut's Basketball team between 1988 and 1992. During my tenure with the team, I had some interesting conversations with Coach Jim Calhoun. While I was coaching, I was also a doctoral student and began to feel confident about my understanding of sports performance. Coach Calhoun and I had a good relationship and we started speaking about the pregame meal. He really wasn't interested in any change and we continued to discuss this for a couple of pregame meals. It is important to understand that Coach Calhoun, who eventually was elected to the Basketball Hall-of-Fame, had a master's degree in psychology and made use of it on a daily basis to motivate his players and staff. He began to explain that on our team there are a number of players who were high school basketball player of the year in their state. Each of those players was the best basketball player from wherever they came from. They averaged 40 points a game, and before each game they had a Big Mac and cheese. Do you really believe that if they had a more appropriate pregame meal, they would have scored 41? He remarked that the most important thing they need to eat is what makes them feel good. I never forgot that lesson. It put the question of the pregame meal or any issue with nutrition in an appropriate context. When I was coaching professional basketball in Israel, we played in the European Championship League and had four former NBA players on our team. Whenever we were in Europe, I was responsible for the pregame meal (we did not have a nutritionist). The first thing I did was asked the players what they preferred to eat and spoke with the chefs at every hotel we stayed at to ensure that the players had the meal that made them feel good. However, during our travel and training during the season, when players began to complain about fatigue or other issues, it was then that the discussion of possible changes to their diet became effective. Those discussions proved to be very helpful. The takeaway from this story is that science is important, but diet is very personal for players and many times small changes are made as the result of continued discussion. Education of the athlete is key! Provide them the knowledge and guide them to the correct choice.

One of the biggest misconceptions in sport nutrition is that it has any relation to athletic ability. It does not. It has absolutely no relationship to football playing ability. It will not differentiate between different levels of performance, nor between starters and nonstarters. It may, however, provide a potential reason why potential was not fulfilled. It may explain why fatigue set in early, it may explain why recovery was inadequate, or why a player had to come off the field for gastrointestinal distress. The value of appropriate nutrition is to allow the player to maintain a high level of training. For athletes to maintain a high level of training, they need to have an energy intake that equals their energy expenditure. The nutritional requirements for an athlete are much different than the general population. Decision based on recommendations made for nonathletes would not be very helpful. In fact, recommendations need to be specific to the needs of the specific athlete.

There are six classes of nutrients that are required for the energy and health needs of all athletes, including the football player: carbohydrates, fats, proteins, vitamins, minerals, and water. Carbohydrates, fats, and proteins are macronutrients and are the principal compounds that make up our food and provide energy for our bodies. Vitamins and minerals have important roles in energy production and are involved in bone health and immune function. However, they provide no direct source of energy. Water may be the most important nutrient available. It is needed for nutrient transport, waste removal, body cooling, and most other body reactions.

Importance of Macronutrient Intake in Football Performance

Energy is produced from three sources. The phosphagen energy system has sufficient energy to fuel high-intensity exercise for up to 30 s, while the glycolytic energy system is the primary energy system fueling high-intensity exercise for 1–3 min (Hoffman, 2014). The phosphagen energy system requires 3 min to fully rephosphorylate adenosine diphosphate (ADP) to adenosine triphosphate (ATP) via creatine phosphate. The glycolytic energy system breaks down carbohydrate to produce 2–3 ATP. Both the phosphagen and glycolytic energy systems do not utilize oxygen and are termed anaerobic. The oxidative energy system does require oxygen, and it is considered to be aerobic. The aerobic energy system is the most efficient in regard to fuel as it primarily uses fat. However, it can do so only in the presence of carbohydrate. The oxidation of fat during prolonged exercise depends on Krebs cycle intermediates that are produced from the breakdown of carbohydrate during the process of glycolysis. When both muscle and liver glycogen stores are depleted, the ability to provide a sufficient amount of the Krebs cycle intermediates is drastically reduced. Although a metabolic profile of the game of football has yet to be scientifically examined, the repetitive high-intensity nature of the game (see Chapter 1) makes football a classic anaerobic strength/power sport. As such, it will rely primarily on carbohydrates as its primary fuel source. However, it is important to understand that all three energy systems are always active; the intensity of the activity determines which is the predominant energy system.

Importance of Carbohydrates

There are several types of carbohydrates that are separated on the basis of their size. Monosaccharides are the simplest form of carbohydrate. They consist of a single-unit sugar molecule such as glucose, fructose, and galactose. Disaccharides are a two-unit sugar molecule such as sucrose (table sugar), maltose (grain sugar), and lactose (milk sugar). Both mono- and disaccharides are considered simple sugars and are a good source of quick energy. Simple carbohydrates are found in natural foods such as fruits (fresh, dried, and juices) and vegetables, as well as in processed foods such as candy and soft drinks. Carbohydrates that contain more than two-unit sugar molecules are termed polysaccharides and are considered complex carbohydrates. Common polysaccharides include starch and glycogen, which is made up primarily of chains of glucose molecules. The bonds that bind the individual carbohydrate units of a complex carbohydrate may be either digestible (such as those found in potatoes, pasta, bread, and beans) or indigestible. Indigestible polysaccharides are known as fiber and are common in some grains, fruits, and vegetables.

The consumption of simple carbohydrates results in a relatively fast increase in glucose concentrations in the blood. This stimulates an insulin response that moves glucose from the blood into muscle, where it can be used for immediate energy or stored for later use. Carbohydrates that are not used immediately are stored in skeletal muscle and/or liver as glycogen. Having full glycogen storage depots is critical for fueling athletic performance. However, if the body's glycogen stores are not full, it may be the reason for earlier onset of fatigue during a practice or competition. However, if glycogen stores are completely full, the excess carbohydrate is converted to fat and stored in adipose sites around the body.

During football practice or competition, muscle glycogen is the primary energy source. As glucose uptake by the active muscle increases, the liver needs to increase the rate at which it breaks down stored glycogen. Unfortunately, the glycogen content of the liver is limited, and the ability of the liver to produce glucose from other substrates (e.g., amino acids) cannot be performed rapidly, thus blood glucose levels decrease. Fatigue quickly sets in as glycogen stores in muscle are reduced. The body does not have the ability to use glycogen reserves from inactive muscles to fuel active muscles. This is related to the lack of the enzyme phosphatase within skeletal muscle. This enzyme is present in the liver, thereby permitting glucose to leave the liver and be transported to exercising muscle. Muscle glycogen depletion is dependent on several factors, including exercise intensity, physical condition, mode of exercise, environmental temperature, and diet (Costill, 1988). When glycogen stores are depressed to very low levels, the intensity of exercise must be reduced to cause a greater reliance on stored fat to fuel muscle activity.

This is the primary reason why much effort has been devoted to maximizing carbohydrate stores within muscle and the liver. Normal muscle glycogen content is approximately 100 mmol·kg^{-1} wet weight for individuals fed a normal carbohydrate diet (55% of total calories); however, when fed a carbohydrate-rich diet (60–70% of total calories) for three days, muscle glycogen content was doubled (Bergstrom et al., 1967). This procedure is known as glycogen loading, and it is a widely used practice for endurance athletes before competition, but its concept can be applied to other athletes, including football players.

Importance of Fats

Fats are a highly concentrated fuel that exists in the body in several forms. The most common form of fat is triglyceride, which is composed of three fatty acids and a glycerol molecule. Another common fat is cholesterol. Fats have several important functions in the body. They provide up to 70% of total energy during rest, support and cushion vital organs, are essential components of cell membranes and nerve fibers, serve as a precursor for steroid hormones, store and transport fat-soluble vitamins, and serve as an insulator to preserve body heat (Hoffman, 2014). The basic unit of fat is the fatty acid, which is also the part of fat that is used for energy production. The two primary fuels that are used to provide energy for muscular activity are carbohydrates and fats. As discussed earlier, the amount of carbohydrate available for energy is limited. Fats, however, have unlimited availability. During an actual football game, high-intensity movements will be fueled primarily through the anaerobic energy system. However, depending upon the position, only 3.8–17.6% of the distance covered during a game will be performed at high intensity or higher (Wellman et al., 2016). The rest of the distance covered during a game will be performed at lower levels of intensity. During these lower levels of intensity, the energy needs of the muscle will likely be met by triglycerides from within the muscle itself and by free fatty acids. Free fatty acids are released from adipose sites around the body and bind to the protein albumin in the blood for transport to the active muscle. The breakdown of fat in peripheral adipocytes (e.g., lipolysis) likely provides the predominant source of energy between plays (jogging back to the huddle and to the line of scrimmage).

The increase in lipolysis (breakdown of triglycerides into free fatty acids) is a result of sympathetic neural stimulation, which is activated by reduced blood glucose levels and also by a stimulatory or anticipatory effect of the game (Hoffman, 2005). The sympathetic hormone norepinephrine binds to its receptor site on the adipose tissue, stimulating activation of the enzyme lipase, which regulates the breakdown of triglycerides into free fatty acids (Hoffman, 2005). The glycerol molecule diffuses out of the adipose tissue and is used for gluconeogenesis in the liver, providing another mechanism of increasing glucose content (Bjorntorp, 1991). The free fatty acids bind to albumin and are transported to the muscle or other end organs to be used for energy.

Importance of Protein

Proteins are nitrogen-containing substances that are formed by amino acids. They are the major structural component of muscle and other tissues in the body. They are also used in the production of hormones, enzymes, and hemoglobin. Proteins can also be used as energy; however, this is not their primary role, and it is used only as a final resort. For proteins to be utilized, they must be broken down into their simplest form: amino acids. There have been 20 amino acids identified that are needed for human growth and metabolism. Eleven of these amino acids are nonessential, meaning that our body can synthesize them, and they do not need to be consumed in the diet. However, the remaining nine amino acids are essential, meaning our body cannot produce them, and they must be consumed in our diet. Absence of any of these essential amino acids from our diet prevents the production of certain proteins that may compromise tissue growth or repair. If the protein portion of the food contains all of the essential amino acids, the protein is called a complete protein. Meats, fish, eggs, and milk are the best sources for complete proteins (Hoffman and Falvo, 2004d). Proteins from plant and grain sources do not supply all of the essential amino acids and are described as incomplete proteins. Thus, for vegetarians to receive all of the essential amino acids, they need to combine proteins from several different plant and grain sources.

The primary role of dietary protein is to stimulate various anabolic processes within the body. However, if carbohydrate stores are depleted, then protein can become a major source of energy. In contrast to carbohydrate and fat, there is no storage depot for protein in the body. The body's skeletal muscle mass is considered the emergency source of protein, and is the reason for muscle atrophy in calorie-restricted diets. During the protein degradation process, the nitrogen molecule is removed from the amino acid through the enzymatic process of transamination and then attached to other compounds. The carbon skeleton of the amino acid can then be metabolized for use as energy, and the nitrogen molecule is excreted. When the body excretes more nitrogen than it consumes, it is said to be in a negative nitrogen balance, indicating that catabolic processes are occurring within the muscle, but if nitrogen intake exceeds nitrogen excretion, the body is in a positive nitrogen balance and anabolic processes are likely predominating. A catabolic state is not conducive for muscle development or enhanced recovery. Thus, it becomes very important to consume a sufficient amount of carbohydrate to reduce protein degradation and maintain a positive nitrogen balance. For athletes, such as the football player, whose training programs are focused on muscle size and strength development, the use of a restricted carbohydrate diet may have severe negative consequences on growth and strength improvements.

The football player as a strength/power athlete requires more protein than recreational or endurance athletes. Resistance exercise is a potent stimulator of muscle protein synthesis, and results in a greater protein accretion than protein degradation (Phillips et al., 1997). However, protein ingestion following resistance exercise augments muscle protein synthesis to a greater extent than resistance exercise alone (Miller et al., 2003; Tipton et al., 1999). Although resistance exercise and protein intake can increase muscle protein synthesis by themselves, the combination of the two provides an augmented response in promoting protein synthesis.

It has been well-accepted that strength/power athletes have a greater daily protein requirement than other athletes and the sedentary adult population (Jäger et al., 2017). A daily protein intake ranging from 1.4 to 2.0 g·kg·day^{-1} is recommended. However, there are several reports that higher daily intakes can be beneficial. In one of the few studies on protein consumption and college football players, the effect of protein intake on lean body mass (LBM) and maximal (1RM) strength was examined (Hoffman et al., 2006b). Players completed dietary recalls throughout the 12-week program. At the conclusion of the off-season program, the players were stratified into one of three groups depending upon their average protein intake. One group consisted of athletes that consumed a daily protein intake below recommended levels (BRL, 1.2 g·kg·day^{-1}), another group consumed a daily protein intake at recommended levels (RL, 1.7 g·kg·day^{-1}), and the final group were athletes who consumed protein at or above recommended levels (ARL, 2.4 g·kg·day^{-1}). Changes in 1RM squat and bench press can be observed in Figure 5.1. No significant differences were noted between the groups in the change (Δ) in LBM. The Δ change in LBM for BRL, RL, and ARL was -0.1 ± 1.6 kg, 0.8 ± 1.5 kg, and 1.1 ± 2.2 kg, respectively. Greater gains in strength were seen in ARL for both the bench press (8.7%) and squat exercises (21.7%) compared to BRL (6.9% and 8.0%, respectively) and RL (7.1% and 12.1%, respectively), but only the Δ 1RM squat strength in ARL was significantly greater than BRL. In a subsequent study on college football players, daily protein intakes of 2 g·kg·day^{-1} for 12 weeks during an off-season conditioning program resulted in significantly greater gains in squat strength compared to the players consuming 1.2 g·kg·day^{-1} (Hoffman et al., 2007).

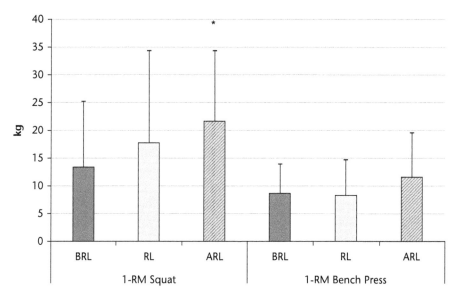

FIGURE 5.1 The Effect of Protein Consumption and Changes in 1RM Squat and Bench Press in College Football Players.

★ = significantly different from BRL and RL; BRL = below recommended levels; RL = recommended levels; ARL = above recommended levels. Data are reported as mean ± SD.

Source: Data from Hoffman et al., 2006b.

A more recent study has examined whether a super high daily intake provided any greater benefit (Antonio et al., 2016). Antonio and colleagues (2016) examined two different daily protein intake groups (2.3 and 3.4 g·kg·day^{-1}) during an eight-week resistance training program (five-day per week split routine) in resistance-trained men and women. Although these were not competitive football players, it does provide some understanding of the potential effect of very high protein intakes. Results revealed no further advantage in strength gains, but significantly greater losses were seen in fat mass in the high protein group.

How Much Protein Can Be Consumed per Ingestion?

An important question regarding protein intake relates to how much protein an athlete can consume per ingestion. Moore and colleagues (2009) examined postexercise protein drinks containing 0, 5, 10, 20, or 40 g of protein following an acute bout of resistance exercise. Results indicated that muscle protein synthesis can continue to increase with protein consumption amounts up to 20 g. No further increase in protein synthesis was seen with the 40 g dose. A subsequent study by the same investigative team examined the pattern of protein intake following resistance exercise (Moore et al., 2012). Resistance-trained men were provided three different dosing patterns: pulse (8 × 10 g of protein every 1.5 h), intermediate (4 × 20 g of protein every 3 h), and bolus (2 × 40 g every 6 h). It was reported that the pulse pattern of ingestion resulted in a significantly greater protein turnover than the bolus pattern (~19%, $p < 0.05$) with a trend toward being greater than intermediate (~9%, $p = 0.08$). Rates of protein synthesis were 32% and 19% greater, and rates of protein breakdown were 51% and 57% greater for the pulse pattern of protein intake compared to both intermediate and bolus patterns, respectively ($p < 0.05$). No differences were noted between intermediate and bolus in protein synthesis or protein breakdown. The results of these studies indicated that there may be an upper limit regarding how much protein can be consumed at a single sitting and that the pattern of protein ingestion favors repeated ingestion of a moderate amount of protein. However, considering that these studies were not conducted in football players and were not performed at a relative dose, it is likely that linemen may benefit from larger doses. However, the repeated ingestion times would likely remain effective for those athletes as well.

Is There a Benefit of Nutrient Timing in Football Players?

One of the more interesting areas of research within sport nutrition has been in nutrient timing. The ingestion of protein at specific times surrounding a workout does appear to have a significant impact on maximizing skeletal muscle adaptation during resistance training programs (Jäger et al., 2017; Kerksick, 2017), and it may also be beneficial in enhancing muscular recovery in trained athletes following an acute exercise session (Hoffman et al., 2010). These effects appear to be related to an enhanced delivery of protein to exercising muscle providing immediate availability of nutrients at the workouts conclusion. The greater muscle protein synthesis immediately following the workout is thought to enhance skeletal muscle adaptation and/or recovery resulting from a heightened muscle sensitivity from the exercise stimulus. Evidence is compelling regarding the importance of ingesting protein immediately before and/or after a training session. Most studies have actually compared feedings surrounding the workout to morning and evening ingestion times (Jäger et al., 2017). However, only one of the studies published has actually examined the effect of nutrient timing in football players during off-season conditioning (Hoffman et al., 2009b). In this study, the football team was divided into three groups: a.m./p.m. – protein feedings in morning and evening; pre/post – protein feedings before and after each workout; a control (CTR) group – no protein feedings except what they consumed with their meals. All three groups consumed the recommended daily amount of protein per day (2.3 g·kg·day^{-1}, 2.2 g·kg·day^{-1}, and 1.7 g·kg·day^{-1} in a.m./p.m., pre/post, and CTR, respectively). The study was ten weeks in duration. At the end of the study, it was observed that all groups remained in a positive nitrogen balance, and all three groups experienced significant improvements in 1-repetition maximum (1RM) squat strength. However, only the am/pm and Pre/Post groups significantly increased 1RM bench press. Although the evidence regarding protein timing was not supported by this study, it is possible that the type of protein used (collagen protein) may not have been ideal to influence performance gains, and the ten-week study duration may not have been of sufficient duration to stimulate strength changes in an experienced group of strength/power athletes.

Evidence is more convincing for the acute effects regarding protein timing and competitive athlete. On January 24 and 25, 2011, 13 members of the University of Iowa's football team were hospitalized for rhabdomyolysis. During the first practice back from winter break players were required to perform 100 repetitions in the squat exercise with 50% of the highest weight lifted by each player at his last assessment (approximately 6 months previous). Players were allowed to take as much time as they needed to complete the 100 repetitions, but each player was timed and most players viewed the squats as a competition. According to the investigation, players who were not diagnosed with rhabdomyolysis were more likely to report that they drank protein shakes after the workouts and that they drank protein shakes on more of the days after the workouts than were players who were hospitalized with rhabdomyolysis (Drake et al., 2011). This unfortunate incident highlighted the importance of protein ingestion following the workout and its potential impact on recovery.

In addition to protein timing, there is evidence that there is a greater sensitivity regarding carbohydrate ingestion and glycogen replenishment shortly after a workout/practice. Considering the importance of carbohydrates in refueling exercise, this is very important in regard to maximizing recovery. Greater insulin sensitivity postexercise maximizes the utilization of high glycemic carbohydrates. Delay in carbohydrate ingestion by 2 h may reduce glycogen resynthesis by ~50% (Ivy et al., 1988). To help determine the appropriate carbohydrate to consume a glycemic index was developed to help classify food on their acute glycemic impact (Burke et al., 1998). Foods with a high glycemic index will be digested quickly and raise blood glucose levels fairly rapidly. Examples of foods with a high glycemic index are baked potato, rice cakes, waffles, and instant rice. Foods with a lower glycemic index will take longer to be digested. Examples of such foods include nuts, fruits, dairy products, and pasta.

What Are the Dietary Habits of Football Players?

There are a limited number of studies that have examined the dietary intake habits of football players: A bit surprising considering the vast number of nutritionists that are now working with teams. One of the first studies that published the energy needs of football players suggested that daily caloric intake needs to range between 4,000 and 5,300 kcal (Short and Short, 1983). Cole and colleagues (2005) examining NCAA Division I football players reported that the average energy intake was 3,288 kcal per day, with 392 g of carbohydrate, 169 g of protein (~1.54 g·kg^{-1}), and 103 g of fat. These results were similar to that reported in NCAA Division III athletes, but the daily protein content was slightly lower (Hoffman et al., 2006b). It should be noted that no mention of a nutritionist or training table that is often part of Division I programs was made. Interestingly, when players were asked who they relied upon for dietary education, only 5% of these players indicated a nutritionist. These results do suggest that the nutritionist has an important role in educating the athlete on proper dietary habits. A later study on NCAA Division I athletes whose dietary habits were followed for eight weeks indicated that their caloric intake increased from 3,518 ± 849 kcal to 5,115 ± 2,391 kcal (Kirwan et al., 2012). In addition, the amount of carbohydrates and protein consumed daily increased 82% and 29%, respectively, from beginning to end of off-season training. Fat consumption decreased 9%. Relative protein intake averaged 1.8 g·kg^{-1} throughout the off-season program. The use of a sport nutrition did appear to assist the athletes in better monitoring their nutrient intake.

The lack of knowledge of appropriate nutritional guidelines is an issue that has been raised by several investigations of both NCAA Division I and III football players (Abbey et al., 2017; Werner et al., 2020). Poor knowledge can lead to athletes formulating bad nutritional choices that can impede recovery from exercise, increase risk for injury, and possibly prevent them from reaching their full potential. Programs should consider having someone on staff, whether a nutritionist or sport scientist to provide consulting on dietary habits.

Importance of Micronutrient Intake in Football Performance

Vitamins and minerals are needed by cells to perform specific functions that promote growth and maintain health. Most vitamins have a role in athletic performance. Their relevance is likely related to their function in energy metabolism and muscle growth. Many athletes, concerned that their high-intensity workouts require a greater vitamin intake, have made vitamin supplements the most popular supplement to purchase (Hoffman, 2019a). However, research has been unable to support any need for vitamin supplementation, especially for athletes competing in a power sport such as football (Hoffman, 2014). It appears that the higher caloric intakes of these athletes more than compensates for any increase in vitamin mineral requirements caused by high-intensity training. However, vitamin and mineral supplementation may prove to be beneficial for athletes who do not have a well-balanced diet or are on a calorie-restricted diet.

Studies have shown promising results in the ability of vitamin supplementation and other micronutrients to serve as antioxidants. Common antioxidants include vitamins C and E, selenium, β-carotene, and coenzyme Q10 (Arroyo and Jajtner, 2019). Additionally, polyphenols are the most plentiful antioxidant in the diet and are common in many plant-based foods and beverages, such as fruits, tea, and coffee. Regardless of the type of polyphenol or antioxidant consumed, one of the primary functions for these micronutrients is to help maintain the oxidative balance within the body (Arroyo and Jajtner, 2019). An increase in reactive oxygen species (ROS) is often observed following intense physical activity. ROS can alter cell integrity and function, and contribute to muscle damage, leading to fatigue, inflammation, and illness; however, within physiological levels, ROS can also promote important training adaptations by acting as signaling molecules that regulate growth, proliferation, and differentiation (Gomes et al., 2012; Powers et al., 2011).

The only vitamin or mineral that has been examined to any extent in football players is vitamin D. Vitamin D acts as a precursor steroid for several biological processes, including bone metabolism, protein synthesis, and muscle function (Arroyo and Jajtner, 2019; Hoffman, 2014). Vitamin D is not a vitamin in its usual sense, but rather behaves similar to steroid hormones. Deficiency in vitamin D is associated with muscle weakness and bone loss. Examination of elite college football players who were invited to the NFL combine were reported to have inadequate vitamin D levels, which was associated with a history of lower extremity muscle strain and core muscle injury (Rebolledo et al., 2018). Vitamin D insufficiency has recently been reported in college football players (Sun et al., 2019), but no discussion regarding its effect on performance or risk of injury was provided.

Importance of Hydration in Football Performance

Water is essential for human life and provides the medium for all biochemical reactions that occur within the body. It is critical for maintaining cardiovascular function and thermoregulation by preserving blood volume. Water constitutes approximately 60% of body mass. Approximately two-thirds of the water in our body is found within our cells (i.e., intracellular fluid), and the remaining fluid is found in various compartments outside of the cell (i.e., extracellular fluid). Extracellular fluid includes the fluid surrounding the cells (interstitial fluid), blood plasma, lymph, and other bodily fluids. Water is second only to oxygen in the necessity for maintaining life. To provide some perspective on the importance of water, humans can withstand a 40% loss in body mass from starvation, but a 9–12% loss of body mass from fluid can be fatal. Considering the importance of water in normal physiological function, it is no surprise that water also has a significant role in maintaining exercise performance. One of its primary roles is to help dissipate metabolic heat during exercise to maintain thermal homeostasis. As discussed in Chapter 2, heat dissipation is primarily accomplished through evaporative cooling (i.e., sweating), which can result in a large loss in water. If fluid intake does not match body water loss, the body is said to be dehydrating, meaning that a body water deficit is occurring. A state of hypohydration (an existing body water deficit) has significant effects on both physiological function and the ability to perform exercise.

A situation of dehydration has significant implications for both cardiovascular and thermoregulatory functions. A reduction in plasma volume results in less blood being available to both exercising muscle and the skin. This will cause a reduction in stroke volume and an

TABLE 5.1 Physiological Effects and Potential Warning Signs of Dehydration

	Body Water Deficit (%)				
	0–2	2–4	4–6	6–8	8–12
Physiological effect	↑ Core temperature	• ↓ Plasma volume • ↓ Intracellular fluid content • ↓ Stroke volume • ↓ Blood flow to skin and muscle • ↓ Heart rate	• ↓ Sweat rate	• ↓ Urine acidity • ↓ Protein in urine • ↓ Blood flow to kidney	–
Warning sign	None	• Thirst • Verbal complaints • Some discomfort	• Flushed skin • Apathy • Clear loss of muscle endurance impatience • Muscle spasms and muscle cramps • Tingling sensation in arms, back, and neck	• Headache • Cotton mouth • Dizziness • Shortness of breath • Indistinct speech	• Swollen tongue • Spasticity • Delirium

Source: Adapted from Armstrong, 1988 and Hoffman, 2014.

elevation in heart rate to maintain normal blood flow. However, depending on the magnitude of the body water deficit, the increase in heart rate may not be sufficient to fully compensate for the lower stroke volume (Armstrong, 2000). A body water deficit can also impair thermoregulation, the severity of which depends on the magnitude of hypohydration. As the body water deficit increases, the ability to dissipate heat will be reduced. This will result in a decrease in both sweating rate and blood flow to the skin (Sawka and Pandolf, 1990). Table 5.1 depicts the physiological effects and potential warning signs of dehydration. As dehydration reaches 5% of body weight, the health of the athlete may become compromised, and at a 9% body water deficit, physiological systems may become impaired.

Performance Effects From Hypohydration

Changes to both cardiovascular and thermoregulatory function during dehydration could have a profound effect on exercise performance. Although much work has been done on endurance performance, fewer investigations have focused on anaerobic sports, specifically football. Performance changes are associated with the magnitude of the body water deficit. Most studies examining the effect of dehydration on anaerobic exercise performance have been conducted on wrestlers who reduce weight quickly to compete at a given weight class. These studies have shown that strength, anaerobic power, and anaerobic capacity are generally not affected by a body mass deficit of up to 5%, as long as the duration of high-intensity activity is less than

40 s (for a complete review, see Hoffman, 2014). However, these studies are not relevant or comparable to a football game. In studies examining longer duration exercise, protocols with a hypohydration stress, decreases in anaerobic power and capacity, have been reported (Horswill et al., 1990; Webster et al., 1990). As duration of anaerobic activity increases, the strain of hypohydration does appear to negatively affect performance.

There have been only a limited number of studies that have been conducted examining the effects of dehydration in sports that rely on intermittent bouts of high-intensity exercise over a relatively long duration. In such sports (e.g., basketball, football, and hockey), athletes do not voluntarily dehydrate to compete at a lighter weight class. Rather, dehydration occurs because fluid intake during the actual game was not sufficient. When anaerobic power needs to be maintained over a moderate duration of time (e.g., 30–60 min), a body water deficit may hinder such performance. In a study examining the effect of fluid restriction on anaerobic power and skill performance during a simulated basketball game, fluid restriction during the 40-min game resulted in an average body water deficit of 1.9% (Hoffman et al., 1995). No significant changes were noted in vertical jump height, anaerobic power, or shooting performance. However, an 8% decrease in shooting percentage (p > 0.05) was reported when subjects were dehydrated. This calculated to result in a possible six-point deficit (average number of shots in a game/ calculated shooting %) during a game. Although this did not have statistical significance, it had a tremendous practical impact. A six-point difference can easily affect the outcome of a game. The results of this study suggested that even at low levels of dehydration, in which the athlete may not perceive thirst, performance in activities that require fine motor control may be impaired. Previously it has been demonstrated that motor unit recruitment patterns and muscle contraction capabilities may be reduced because of elevated body temperatures and electrolyte imbalances occurring from the combined exercise and hydration stress (Sjogaard, 1986). In a subsequent study conducted 17 years later in a NCAA Division I women's competitive basketball game, a 2.3% loss in body mass was associated with an impaired shooting percentage and reaction time, compared to a contest in which the women were permitted to drink ad libitum (Hoffman et al., 2012). Interesting, no differences were noted in the change in vertical jump power during either trial.

One of the most important aspects of practice and game preparation for football is to provide the opportunity for players to rehydrate as often as possible. If the football player, or any athlete, relies only on thirst as an indicator to drink, he will undoubtedly perform in a dehydrated condition. The sensation of thirst does not occur until a body water deficit reaches approximately 2%. Even at this magnitude of hypohydration, physiological changes are apparent and performance decrements can be seen. In football, the ability to rehydrate is relatively easy compared to many other sports. As soon as the player comes off the field, they should be strongly encouraged to rehydrate. There should be an accessible table or water station on the sidelines of each game, and water stations available in practice. Even when fluid is available, athletes seldom consume more than 0.5 $L \cdot h^{-1}$ (Noakes, 1993). Thus, athletes need to adopt several strategies to maintain a normal body fluid balance. Several recommendations for maintaining fluid balance are listed in Table 5.2.

The ability of football players to rehydrate has been questioned by several investigations. In a study on NCAA Division II football players, athletes were monitored for changes in body mass before and after every practice during the first eight days of training camp that included two practice sessions per day (Godek et al., 2005). Figure 5.2 details the day-to-day change in body mass prior to practice and post-second practice. It is very clear that thirst was insufficient to guide the athlete to rehydrate adequately. Sweat rates were reported to be $2 L \times h^{-1}$ and with 4.5 h of practice per day, the investigators estimated that the football players were losing approximately

TABLE 5.2 Recommendations for Maintaining Fluid Balance in Football Practice and Competitions

General strategies	• Ingested fluids should be between 59°F and 72°F (15°C and 22°C) and flavored to enhance palatability to promote maximal fluid replacement • Athletes should weigh themselves after each practice and game and replace all lost fluid. The athlete should rehydrate 1 L for each kg of body weight lost • Changes in body weight and urine color; urine-specific gravity are indicators of hydration status and should be routinely examined
Pregame or practice hydration strategies	• Drink 0.5 L of water 2 h before exercise to promote adequate hydration and allow for excretion of excess fluid • Athlete should then drink an additional 200–300 ml of fluid 10–20 min prior to exercise
During game or practice hydration strategies	• Forced hydration should be practiced (drinking even when the thirst sensation is absent) during every time-out or stoppage of play during practice or a game to prevent physiological and performance impairments • Athlete should optimize, not maximize fluid intake without overhydrating • Electrolyte drinks have not been proven to delay fatigue during exercise less than 3–4 h in duration. However, glucose-electrolyte drinks may delay fatigue in exercise of shorter duration
Postexercise hydration strategies	• Fluids consumed following exercise can be with or without carbohydrates and electrolytes. However, water alone may not be the optimal rehydration beverage because it decreases osmolality (a measure of solute concentration) limiting the urge to drink and may increase urine output • Because replacement of expended glycogen stores is also a postexercise goal, the rehydration solution should contain carbohydrates. Carbohydrates may also help to improve the intestinal absorption of sodium and water. • Some team physicians may use an intravenous fluid infusion to rehydrate athletes at half time of a contest. However, no performance differences between infusion and normal oral rehydration techniques when rehydration and rest periods ranged from 20 to 75 min between exercise sessions (Casa et al., 2012). During a 15-min half-time period, this rehydration strategy is debatable

Source: Adapted from Hoffman, 2014.

9 L of sweat per day. The large daily volumes of sweat loss that was replaced with hypotonic fluids (water only) appeared to promote sodium dilution. This was confirmed in urinary sodium and potassium changes. By the end of the eight-day study, urinary excretions of both sodium and potassium were significantly lowered, reflecting kidney conservation of electrolytes. Plasma volume increased up to 14% by days 6 and 8 of the study, reflecting the increased conservation of sodium attempting to maintain plasma volume. An important finding from the study was the effect of water temperature on rehydration. The players lost 24.3% (0.5 kg) more weight when they drank the warmer fountain water compared to drinking cold water. Others have reported average sweat rates of college football players of 1.5 L·h^{-1} (Barnes et al., 2019).

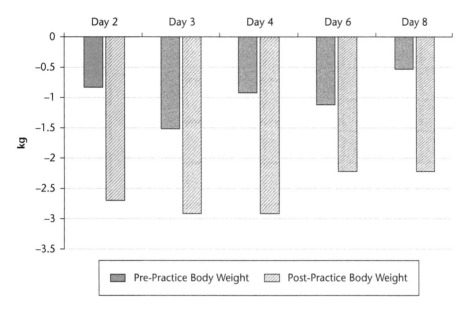

FIGURE 5.2 Changes in Pre-Practice and Post-Practice Body Weights in College Football Players. *Source:* Data from Godek et al., 2005.

In a subsequent study, Godek and colleagues (2008) compared hydration practices between NFL linemen and skill position players. As expected, linemen were taller, heavier, and had a greater body surface area (BSA) than the skill position players. However, the BSA-to-mass ratio was lower in the linemen. Sweat rate was significantly greater in linemen (2.4 ± 0.5 L·h⁻¹) than skill position players (1.4 ± 0.6 L·h⁻¹). When adjusted for BSA, linemen had a 32.5% greater sweat rate (p = 0.06) than skill position players (0.89 ± 0.22 L·h⁻¹ versus 0.67 ± 0.33 L·h⁻¹, respectively). Fluid consumption rate was also greater in linemen than in skill position players (1.3 ± 0.3 L·h⁻¹ versus 0.7 ± 0.4 L·h⁻¹, respectively), and total fluid intake was also significantly greater in linemen than skill position players (2.0 ± 0.8 L·h⁻¹ versus 1.2 ± 0.8 L·h⁻¹, respectively). Percent weight loss during practices were nearly identical between linemen (21.2 ± 0.8 %) and skill position players (21.1 ± 0.8%). The results of this study indicated that linemen sweat at a higher rate and lose larger volumes of sweat during practices compared with skill position players. They also consumed more fluids and produced less urine during practices compared with the skill players, and this was likely responsible for the similar loss of percent body weight between the two positions.

A study on rehydration drinking strategies in high school football players during twice-a-day practice in training camp was conducted by Stover and colleagues in 2006. Forty-six players were studied for five days. The mean sweat rate was 0.91 L·h⁻¹ and mean change in body weight during practice was −1.12 ± 0.74%. In regard to rehydration strategy, most players (all but one) chose to use a sports drink versus water only to rehydrate, showing the importance of flavor to entice rehydration. Sweat rates were lower than what had been previously observed in college and professional football players. Despite the lower sweat rate, these athletes were still unable to maintain their body mass during the five-day training camp, indicating a less than optimal rehydration strategy. Subsequent research by others confirmed the inability of high school athletes to adhere to a rehydration strategy to maintain body weight during summer training camp (Yeargin et al., 2010). What was most interesting of this latter study was that despite the athletes' self-perception of consistently good hydration habits, participants replaced most sweat loss during practice but remained hypohydrated throughout the preseason practices suggesting inadequate rehydration habits outside of practice. Thus, when coaches and trainers force hydration, players are able to adequately hydrate, but this practice is not maintained outside the practice field when the external influence is removed.

An important issue that was also raised earlier in this chapter is player knowledge. In a survey examining fluid replacement knowledge of NCAA Division I football players, it was demonstrated that football players specifically lack the basic understanding of appropriate hydration practices (Judge et al., 2016). Again, this highlights the importance of football programs having someone on staff provide this educational service to their athletes.

Popular Nutritional Supplements for Football

The use of dietary supplements among college football players is not well understood. Despite the perception of its popularity, there is limited to no data available regarding supplement use patterns in high school, college, and professional football players. The frequency of supplement use in a variety of populations range from ~50% in adults to ~80% in elite athletes (Hoffman, 2019a), but specific use patterns among football players is lacking. The supplement use pattern among football players is likely on the higher end of the spectrum. Over the past 30 years, the multitude of studies examining the efficacy of various dietary supplements on strength and power performance has provided some very good information to help athletes, coaches, and sport nutritionists have a better understanding of what ingredients may be relevant for the football player. To review every supplement that has been suggested for the football player would require a book by itself, and I highly recommend a recent book published in this area – *Dietary Supplementation in Sport and Exercise, Evidence, Safety and Ergogenic Benefits*, published by Routledge Press – for the reader who wishes to have a more in-depth discussion on various supplements. In this section, I will focus on a handful of the more popular supplements being used by football players: protein, creatine, beta-alanine, and caffeine.

Protein Use in Football Players

Earlier in the chapter, the importance of protein as a macronutrient was discussed. However, the window of adaptation that exists immediately after a workout or perhaps to expedite recovery following practice or postgame would be more efficiently achieved with a protein supplement. The largest benefit supporting the use of protein and amino acid supplementation is the importance that has been placed on the timing of ingestion. As such, the most convenient and efficient method for providing pre-event (pre-practice) or post-event (post-practice) feedings may be through supplementation. There has been plenty written on the benefits of protein supplementation. One of the biggest questions that a player may have is regarding the type of protein to consume. Most protein supplements come as a proprietary blend, meaning there are different types of proteins within the supplement. Two of the most popular protein types are milk proteins called casein and whey. They are commonly used whole proteins found in many protein supplements with different digestive properties. Casein is the predominant milk protein and upon ingestion, it forms a gel or clot in the stomach that makes it slow to digest. As a result, casein provides a sustained, but slow release of amino acids into the bloodstream, sometimes lasting for several hours (Boirie et al., 1997). This provides better nitrogen retention and utilization by the body. Whey protein accounts for 20% of bovine milk (casein accounting for the remainder) that contains high levels of the essential and branched chain amino acids (Hoffman and Falvo, 2004d). Whey protein is the translucent liquid part of milk that remains following the process (coagulation and curd removal) of cheese manufacturing; as a result, it is absorbed into the body much quicker than casein. Both casein and whey are complete proteins, but their amino acid composition is different. Leucine content, which has an important role in muscle protein metabolism, is higher in whey than in casein. Although the total net muscle protein synthesis appears to be similar between the proteins, it is not clear whether the acute elevation seen following whey represents a greater window of opportunity following exercise for enhancing the recovery and remodeling of skeletal muscle. This may have greater relevance regarding the importance of timing. Protein supplementation immediately after a workout/practice/game may be more advantageous to be comprised primarily of whey protein. However, protein supplementation at other times of the day may have greater benefit from a mixed protein or primarily casein.

There has been a tremendous amount of research conducted on protein supplementation, but there appears to be only one study that has examined the effect of protein supplementation in football players. In this one study, 21 NCAA Division III college football players were randomly assigned to either a protein group (proprietary blend of milk protein concentrate, whey protein concentrate, L-glutamine, and dried egg white) or a placebo group (maltodextrin) (Hoffman et al., 2007). The study was conducted during the team's 12-week off-season conditioning program. All players performed the identical four-day per week split routine training program. The daily protein intake for the supplement group was 2.0 ± 0.12 g·kg^{-1} and 1.2 ± 0.12 g·kg^{-1} for the placebo group. Although no significant differences were noted in changes in body mass or LBM, the protein group gained 0.9 ± 1.8 kg and 1.4 ± 1.9 kg, respectively, and the placebo group 0.4 ± 2.0 kg and 0.1 ± 1.4 kg, respectively. Although these differences were not statistically different, the more than 10 fold increase in LBM in the protein group was important. Changes in 1RM bench press and squat can be seen in Figure 5.3. No differences were noted in 1RM bench press, but a significantly greater gain in lower body strength was observed

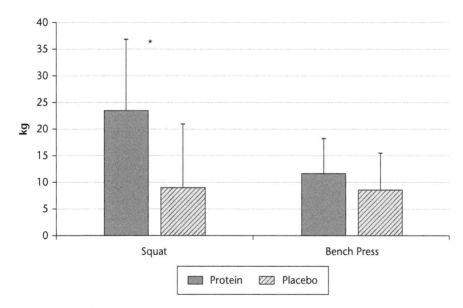

FIGURE 5.3 The Effect of Protein Supplementation on Strength Changes in College Football Players. $\star$ = significant differences between the groups. Data are reported as mean $\pm$ SD.

Source: Data from Hoffman et al., 2007.

in the protein group (14.8%) compared to the placebo group (6.9%). Although no significant changes in 1RM bench press were noted, the protein supplementation group experienced a 9.5% increase in strength, while the placebo group realized only a 6.8% strength improvement.

The protein supplement that has been examined in football players more than any other protein is β-hydroxy-β-methylbutyrate (HMB). HMB is a derivative of the conversion of the amino acid leucine to its metabolite α-ketoisocaproate (Nissen and Abumrad, 1997). Leucine has a well-known anabolic role in muscle by acting as a signaling molecule that stimulates protein synthesis. Nearly 60 g of leucine is required to produce 3 g of HMB, thus supplementing with HMB appears to be a more practical and efficient method of increasing HMB concentrations in skeletal muscle (Gepner et al., 2019; Townsend, 2019). HMB has been widely used as an ergogenic supplement, to increase muscle strength, muscle hypertrophy, and enhance recovery during resistance training (Gepner et al., 2019; Townsend, 2019). The physiological mechanism that underlies these benefits is related to HMB's ability to stimulate muscle protein synthesis and minimize muscle breakdown during periods of stressful training (Eley et al., 2007; Wilkinson et al., 2013).

Kreider and colleagues (2000) were the first investigators to examine the efficacy of HMB in NCAA Division I College football players. They examined 3 g of calcium HMB for 28 days in a placebo-controlled study during the team's winter conditioning program. No significant differences were noted in training volume or body mass changes between the groups. Others were also unable to show any beneficial effect in four weeks of HMB supplementation (3 g of calcium HMB) during off-season training in college football players (Ransone et al., 2003). The results of these studies were not surprising considering that changes in strength for a trained group of strength/power athletes is difficult to achieve in only a four-week study. A subsequent investigation examined whether ten days of HMB supplementation (3 g per day of calcium HMB) could reduce stress and muscle damage associated with twice-a-day training sessions during summer training camp in NCAA Division III football players (Hoffman et al., 2004b). No differences were noted in any of the hormonal or muscle damage markers, suggesting that HMB was not effective to attenuate stress or muscle damage in this short-duration study. The studies of HMB supplementation and football have not proven to be effective. However, this appears to be more of a function of study design and HMB formulation. The use of HMB in its free acid form has proven to be much more effective than the calcium salt form (Townsend, 2019). Further, there has been numerous studies in animal and humans that have demonstrated clear efficacy with HMB (Gepner et al., 2019; Townsend, 2019). Further examination of HMB in football is definitely warranted.

Considering the costs of some protein supplements, a question that may be raised is whether the benefits seen from protein ingestion are better served from a supplement or can similar benefits be achieved from a food source. Milk consumption has been demonstrated to stimulate amino acid uptake by skeletal muscle and result in an increase in net muscle protein synthesis (Elliot et al., 2006). Whole milk appears to be more beneficial than fat-free milk, unless the quantity of fat-free milk consumed is similar in caloric value as whole milk (Elliot et al., 2006). These results demonstrate that a food source such as milk may be suitable for ingestion during recovery, and may be a cheaper and effective alternative to protein supplements. The primary benefit of taking a supplement as a post-workout drink is the ease of preparation and the ability to provide a large intake of protein that is quickly absorbed within the time frame that the exercising tissue is at a heightened sensitivity. A milk machine or refrigerator within the training facility or locker room can provide a cheaper and effective alternative to the costs associated with protein supplementation.

Creatine Use in Football Players

Creatine is one of the most popular supplements for strength/power athletes and one of the most thoroughly examined ergogenic aids. Creatine is a nitrogenous organic compound that is synthesized naturally in the body, primarily within the liver. It can also be consumed in the diet where it is found in both meat and fish. Creatine is stored within skeletal muscle in either its free form or its phosphorylated form (PCr). When it is in its phosphorylated form, it has a critical role in energy metabolism. It acts as a substrate in the formation of adenosine triphosphate (ATP) by rephosphorylating adenosine diphosphate (ADP). This is critical during short-duration, high-intensity exercise. The ability to rapidly rephosphorylate ADP to ATP is dependent upon the enzyme creatine kinase and the availability of PCr within the muscle. As PCr concentrations are lowered, the ability to maintain or perform high-intensity exercise is reduced. This is why creatine is such an important supplement for the football player. During high-intensity, repetitive exercise (such as might be experienced during a football game), PCr concentrations within muscle may approach depletion (Rawson et al., 2019). If muscle PCr concentrations remain elevated, the ability to sustain high-intensity exercise will be maintained. This is the basis behind creatine supplementation.

There have been a number of studies examining creatine supplementation and football. One of the first studies was published by Rick Kreider in 1998. They reported that 28 days of creatine supplementation in NCAA Division I football players resulted in significant gains in LBM, resistance training volume, and sprint and agility performance compared to placebo (Kreider et al., 1998). Bemben and colleagues (2001) provided creatine supplementation (one week of 20 g·day^{-1}, followed by eight-weeks of 5 g·day^{-1}) to NCAA Division I football players in a placebo-controlled, parallel design study with a control group. They reported significantly greater gains in body mass (3.5%) and LBM (3.8%) in the creatine group only. In addition, greater gains were noted in 1RM bench press (5.2%), 1RM squat (8.7%), anaerobic power (19.6%), anaerobic capacity (18.4%), and fatigue rate (−15.9%) in the creatine group. Maximal strength comparison between all three groups from this study can be observed in Figure 5.4. A subsequent study by

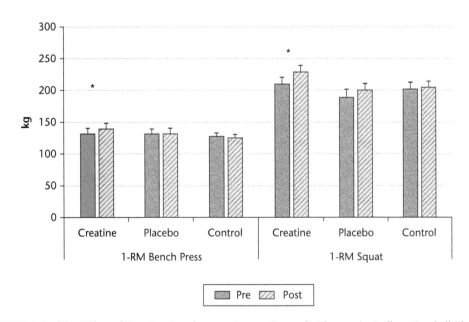

FIGURE 5.4 The Effect of Creatine Supplementation on Strength Changes in College Football Players. ★ = significant differences between the groups; 1RM = one repetition maximum. Data are reported as mean ± SD.

Source: Data from Bemben et al., 2001.

Wilder and colleagues (2002) was unable to demonstrate any significant effect of creatine supplementation in college football players performing a ten-week periodized resistance training program. However, they divided 25 college football players into three groups (low-dose creatine – 3 g·day^{-1}, loading dose – 20 g·day^{-1} for a week followed by 5 g·day^{-1} for the remaining of the study, and a placebo group). The low-dose group experienced a 19 kg improvement in 1RM squat, while the loading dose and placebo group experienced 8.8 g improvements each. These differences were not significant, leading the investigators to conclude that creatine did not provide any further benefit than a periodized resistance training program. Considering that the n size for each group was quite low, it looks like the study was not powered appropriately. Subsequent research examining NCAA Division III football players reported a significant 2.5-fold improvement from placebo in 1RM bench press for creatine (10.5 g·day^{-1}) and a ~20 kg greater improvement in 1RM squat (Hoffman et al., 2006a). Creatine supplementation was also associated with significant increases in resting testosterone concentrations.

β-Alanine Use in Football Players

β-Alanine is considered to be one of the more popular supplements being used by competitive athletes to improve strength/power performance (Saunders and Dolan, 2019). Its efficacy has been summarized in a number of recent reviews (Hoffman et al., 2018; Varanoske et al., 2018). β-Alanine is a nonproteogenic amino acid, and it does not appear to have any ergogenic potential by itself. Once ingested, it combines with histidine within skeletal muscle and other organs to form carnosine. Carnosine is a highly effective intracellular pH buffer, making it ideal to reduce fatigue during high-intensity exercise. β-Alanine is the rate-limiting step in muscle carnosine synthesis (Harris et al., 2006); thus, the primary goal of β-alanine supplementation is to increase carnosine content in skeletal muscle, thereby enhancing intracellular buffering capacity and enabling a greater tolerance of sustained anaerobic activity. It has also been suggested that intramuscular carnosine may also act as a diffusible Ca^{2+}/H^+ exchanger at the level of the sarcomere, augmenting skeletal muscle force production (Swietach et al., 2013). Because carnosine can bind both H^+ and Ca^{2+}, increases of H^+ binding to carnosine may induce Ca^{2+} unloading at the sarcomere, subsequently increasing cross-bridge formation and force production. Additional physiological roles have also been associated with carnosine. Several studies have suggested that carnosine may serve as a neuroprotector (Boldyrev et al., 2010; Hoffman et al., 2018). This is supported by evidence demonstrating carnosine's biological role as an antioxidant and antiglycating and ion-chelating agent (Boldyrev et al., 2004; Kohen et al., 1988; Trombley et al., 2000). Carnosine's antioxidant properties have been demonstrated through its ability to scavenge reactive oxygen species and react directly with superoxide anions and peroxyl radicals in vitro (Boldyrev et al., 2010). High-intensity exercise elicits a significant oxidative stress response, causing inflammation and muscle damage (Packer, 1997). Attenuation of oxidative stress is beneficial to the recovery process and subsequent exercise performance.

There have been several studies examining β-alanine and football players. The first study published compared the combination of β-alanine and creatine to creatine by itself and a placebo (Hoffman et al., 2006a). Thirty-three NCAA Division III college football players were randomized into three groups during the 12-week off-season conditioning program. The combination of β-alanine (3.2 g·day^{-1}) with creatine (10.5 g·day^{-1}) has significantly greater effects on LBM and percent body fat than creatine alone or placebo. This was suggested to be related to the significantly greater training volume observed in the log books of the football players. Simply, the addition of β-alanine improved the quality of the workout for these players. Although strength was significantly improved and significantly greater than placebo for both 1RM bench press and 1RM squat, no differences were noted between the combination of β-alanine with creatine or creatine by itself. It did not appear that the addition of β-alanine has any influence on augmenting strength gains more so than creatine alone. In a second study, β-alanine alone (4.5 g·day^{-1}) was provided for three weeks to college football players prior to preseason training camp (Hoffman et al., 2008b). As later research would confirm, this was not of sufficient dose nor duration to result in significant performance benefits (Hoffman et al., 2018). Football players performed a 60-s Wingate anaerobic power test. This is an extremely fatiguing event that requires maximal effort for the duration of the exam. Results indicated no significant differences in peak power (991 ± 116 and 1,065 ± 172 W), mean power (494 ± 32 and 480 ± 28 W), and total work (29,752 ± 1,913 and 28,789 ± 1,669) between the β-alanine and placebo groups, respectively. However, a trend (p = 0.07) was noted in the rate of fatigue between the two groups favoring β-alanine. In addition, during training camp, subjective feelings of fatigue were significantly lower in the β-alanine group than the placebo group. Finally, examination of the players' log books revealed a significant higher training volume for the bench press exercise in the players supplementing with β-alanine compared to placebo group. Subsequent research provided football players with 4 g·day^{-1} for 8 weeks (Kern and Robinson, 2011). Supplementation with β-alanine appears to have the ability to augment performance and stimulate lean mass accrual in experienced, resistance-trained athletes. The investigators concluded that β-alanine can magnify the expected performance outcomes of training programs.

Caffeine Use in Football Players

Caffeine is one of the most widely used supplements in the world today. It is found in coffee, tea, soft drinks, chocolate, and various other foods. Although caffeine is a central nervous system (CNS) stimulant, its effects are much weaker than those associated with amphetamines. Caffeine is used as an ergogenic aid by both endurance and strength/power athletes. However, the mechanism of action is different. Caffeine is thought to enhance the mobilization of fatty acids from adipose tissue, helping to prolong exercise (Spriet, 1995). The greater use of fat as a primary energy source will slow glycogen depletion and delay fatigue. During short-duration, high-intensity exercise, caffeine is thought to enhance power production by enhancing muscle activation through motor unit recruitment (Warren et al., 2010). In addition, it is also thought to enhance the excitation–contraction coupling associated with neuromuscular transmission and mobilization of intracellular calcium ions from the sarcoplasmic reticulum (Tarnopolsky, 1994). Caffeine is also thought to enhance the kinetics of glycolytic regulatory enzymes such as phosphorylase (Spriet, 1995).

There appears to be a dose–response effect with caffeine supplementation in strength-power performance. The dose that is generally associated with a positive effect of caffeine supplementation is 5–6 mg·kg^{-1}. Thus, for a 90-kg football player, the dose would be approximately 450 mg of caffeine. To put this in some perspective, a generic cup of drip coffee contains between 110 and 150 mg of caffeine (Hoffman, 2014). Energy drinks typically contain between 75 and 174 mg with some exceeding 500 mg (Hoffman, 2019b). Although there is evidence supporting the use of caffeine in enhancing strength, power, and anaerobic activities (see Hoffman, 2014; Wells, 2019), there is much less information regarding caffeine and football. Woolf and colleagues (2009) examined the effects of a moderate dose of caffeine (5 mg·kg^{-1}) on anaerobic performance in highly trained collegiate football players. Participants in the study reported to the laboratory and consumed the caffeine supplement with carbohydrate (0.125 g·kg^{-1}) or carbohydrate only (placebo) and consumed a meal 15 min later. Sixty minutes after consuming the meal, participants performed three assessments: a 40-yard sprint, 20-yard shuttle, and the maximum number of repetitions in a 100 kg bench. Although no significant differences were seen in any of the performance measures between the groups, 59% of the participants decreased time during the 40-yard sprint, 59% decreased time during the 20-yard shuttle, and 47% increased the number of repetitions performed during the bench press while supplementing with caffeine. The investigators suggested that their participants were either caffeine naïve or very low caffeine users, which may have contributed to the results. Another study examining caffeine supplementation in football players recruited 20 NCAA Division I players for a double-blind, cross-over design (participants served as their own controls) (Gwacham and Wagner, 2012). The investigators used a multi-ingredient supplement containing 120 mg of caffeine (approximately 1.2 mg·kg^{-1}) and 200 mg of taurine. Taurine is found in high concentrations in skeletal muscle and is thought to play a role in modulating contractile function and increasing force production by enhancing the accumulation and release of calcium from the sarcoplasmic reticulum. Players performed a running-based anaerobic sprint test, which consisted of six 35-m maximal-effort sprints with 10 s of recovery between each sprint. Results showed no difference in sprint time or anaerobic power between trials (caffeine versus placebo). The low-dose caffeine, regardless of taurine content), was not sufficient to cause any ergogenic effect.

Nutritional Considerations for Practice and Competition

Pre-Practice or Pre-Competition Meal

There is no question that eating a meal is better than practicing or playing a game following a long fast (Rodriguez et al., 2009). Ideally, the meal should be consumed approximately 3–4 h before the event and comprise 200–300 g of carbohydrate. Although there is some debate regarding how close to a practice or game one should eat due to a hypoglycemic response, it is now thought that such a meal may ensure that blood glucose levels remain elevated and prevent feelings of hunger (Hoffman, 2014). A liquid meal close to practice or competition is less likely to cause gastric discomfort. Recommended guidelines for a pre-practice or pre-competition meal are listed in Table 5.3.

TABLE 5.3 Nutritional Recommendations Surrounding Practice and Competition

Event	Recommendations
Pre-practice/competition	• Sufficient in fluid to maintain hydration • Low in fat and fiber to facilitate gastric emptying and gastrointestinal distress • High in carbohydrate to maintain blood glucose and maximize filling of glycogen stores • Moderate in protein intake • Made up of foods familiar to the athlete • Eaten 3–4 h before the game or practice
During practice/competition	• Possible benefit of a high glycemic carbohydrate to maintain blood glucose concentrations
Post-practice/competition	• Consume meal within 2 h of the end of practice or competition • Use high-glycemic carbohydrate • Meal needs to contain sufficient protein (20 g)

In-Practice or Competition Feedings

There is limited data regarding feedings during high-intensity, intermittent exercise such as football. However, if the athlete has an inadequate glycogen supply, they would likely benefit from carbohydrate supplementation during either the practice or competition.

Post-Practice of Competition Meal

The timing of the postexercise/practice or post-competition meal is important. It is generally recommended that a meal be eaten within 2 h of the end of practice or competition (Hoffman, 2014). The closer the meal is to the conclusion of the exercise or competition, the greater the opportunity to maximize glycogen replenishment. The type of carbohydrate may also be important. It is generally recommended that carbohydrates with a high glycemic index be consumed following exercise or competition. Foods with a high glycemic index are digested quickly and raise blood glucose levels fairly rapidly. In addition, the post-practice or competition meal needs to contain sufficient protein (20 g). The primary role of protein consumption is to enhance muscle repair and other anabolic processes within the muscle. It is thought that the interaction of these two nutrients leads to a more anabolic state because of the combined influence of the hormone insulin (Roy et al., 2000).

Summary

This chapter provided a brief understanding of the six nutrient classes and popular supplements that are common to football. It appears that to maintain a high level of performance, football players need to increase their energy intake to a level that equals their high energy expenditures. An increase in caloric expenditure will meet all vitamin and mineral requirements, unless the athlete is on a restricted diet regimen. The football player though does need to ensure that dietary protein consumed per day is close to or exceeds 2.0 $g \cdot kg^{-1}$. The chapter also detailed the importance of rehydration and how specific dietary supplements may be beneficial for the football player.

6

MEDICAL ISSUES ASSOCIATED WITH AMERICAN FOOTBALL

Introduction

Football is considered to be a high-risk sport in regard to injury. On every play there is contact, at times extremely violent. The best way to describe a football game is perhaps as "controlled violence". It is competitive, intense, and requires a special type of person to play this game. Besides the physical attributes discussed in Chapter 4, to be successful in this sport requires a degree of toughness, physicality, teamwork, and perseverance that may be very difficult to measure or quantify. To fully comprehend the rate of injury, one needs to appreciate the desire of these athletes to play through injury, potentially exacerbating its severity. Coaches have preached to players from even as early as *Pop Warner football* to "know the difference between pain and injury – play through the pain but stop when you are injured". Well how is a 12-year-old to know the difference? By the time the player reaches high school or college, this thought process has turned into a habit. In addition, contact sports in general, but especially football, have a limited number of competitions. For the high school or college football players, they may have a maximum of a 40–48 game career. Any game missed is gone forever. Football is a sport that once you stop playing competitively, it is over. There is no recreational football to participate in. The early end to one's career, especially at a young age, makes the thought of missing a game difficult to accept. As such, these players may be willing to take a risk that other athletes may not. Decision-making may not be rational for many of these players. To provide some degree of safety, the medical staff plays an important role in mitigating potential erroneous decisions.

To minimize the extent and magnitude of injury, the National Collegiate Athletic Association (NCAA), National Football League (NFL), and various high school athletic associations, with their medical and coaching committees, over time have made rule changes to minimize risk and enhance player safety. The rules of the game have evolved; techniques taught from a generation ago such as spearing (using your head as the direct point of contact), posting (one blocker engages and the other blocker hits the defender low), head-slaps, bumping receivers down-field, crack-back blocks (receivers turning back to hit a defender in his blind side), horse-collar tackles, etc. are now penalized. These penalties were all created to enhance the safety of the sport. Additional regulations have also been passed to enhance player's safety regarding where and how you can legally hit an opponent. The penalty of "targeting" can result in a disqualification of a player who hits a defenseless opponent. This penalty has created some controversy in that it is usually on a play that for generations of football players would have resulted in cheers. Targeting is defined as a player "taking aim at an opponent for purposes of attacking with forcible contact that goes beyond making a legal tackle or a legal block or playing the ball". This includes actions of *launching* – when a player leaves his feet to attack an opponent by an upward and forward thrust of the body to make forcible contact in the head or neck area. It is also considered targeting if the player is in a *crouch* and then proceeds in an upward and forward thrust to attack with forcible contact at the head or neck area, even though one or both feet are still on the ground. Leading with the helmet, shoulder forearm, fist, hand, or elbow to attack with forcible contact at the head or neck area is also considered targeting. In addition, lowering the head before attacking by initiating forcible contact with the crown of his helmet is also considered targeting. The risk of injury is so great that when the athlete is in such a vulnerable position that not only is a "personal foul" penalty assessed (15 yard loss on the play), but the player can also be ejected from the game, and if the penalty occurs in the second half of the game, the player may be suspended for the first half of his next game as well.

This chapter will focus on the frequency of injury or injury rate and types of injury seen in youth, high school, college, and professional football. Specific discussion will focus on concussion, including risk of occurrence, etiology, symptoms, blood markers of brain injury, and return to play issues. Heat injury was a focus of Chapter 2 and will not be discussed further here. However, it should be acknowledged that it was calculated as part of the injury risk in previous injury surveillance surveys (Dick et al., 2007a). The effect of injury on long-term health, especially in the retired athlete, will be discussed in greater detail in Chapter 7.

Injury Rate

The inherent physicality associated with the game of football creates a natural aphrodisiac for athletes who enjoy the competitive nature of a gladiator sport. It was not surprising to see in a study comparing injury rates in different college sports that football yielded the greatest number of injuries (36.3% of the total injuries reported per year) (Kerr et al., 2015). An average of 47,199 injuries are reported per year in football alone (combined from games and practice sessions), while a total of 130,000 injuries reported on average per year was reported in 25 overall sports encompassing fall, winter, and spring seasons. Interestingly, football was not the top-rated sport in regard to rate of injury (9.2 injuries per 1,000 athlete-exposures), this honor belonged to men's ice hockey that led the way with 9.5 injuries per 1,000-athlete-exposures. However, there are only 386,168 athlete-exposures per year for men's ice hockey, while there are 5,154,055 athlete-exposures per year in college football.

The first in-depth injury surveillance study published in college football appeared in 2007 (Dick et al., 2007b). It comprised a 16-year review (1988–2004) of injury occurrence across all NCAA divisions, an average of 18.8% of schools with football programs participated in the surveillance program. During this 16-year period, the total number of college football players increased from 47,942 to 59,980 (Irick, 2019). This 25% increase in player participation was likely related to the 18% increase in number of NCAA institutions fielding a football team at the NCAA Division I, II, or III level (Dick et al., 2007b). Because injury rates for both games and fall practices did not differ between the divisions, the investigative team decided to pool the data from all three divisions and reported injury rate relative to 1000 athlete-exposures. Each session or game was an exposure. Injuries were reported per practice, per game, or per spring practice. An injury was defined as one that occurred during participation in an organized intercollegiate practice or competition that required medical attention by the team's athletic trainer or physician and resulted in restriction of the player's participation or performance for one or more calendar days beyond the day of injury (Dick et al., 2007a). The injury rate for game and for practice sessions appear in Figure 6.1. The injury risk per game was nine times higher than the practice injury rate (35.9 versus 3.8 injuries per 1,000 exposures, respectively). Although not reported in Figure 6.1, the risk of injury for athletes participating in spring practice was more than twice than seen in fall practice (9.62 versus 3.80 injuries per 1,000 athlete-exposures). This supports the discussion of Chapter 3 regarding the risks associated with spring football practice.

The most common type of injury, its location, and frequency are listed in Table 6.1. The table includes data reported by Dick et al. (2007b). Only injuries that accounted for at least 1% of the total injuries recorded are included in this table. The table provides data from both

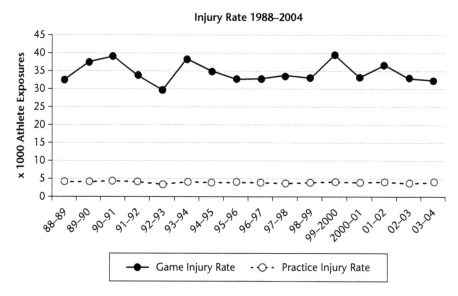

FIGURE 6.1   Injury Rate per 1,000 Athlete-Exposures in Practice and Games.
Source: Data from Dick et al., 2007b.

TABLE 6.1 Most Common Location and Frequency of Injury in 1988/1989–2003/2004 Seasons

% Injury Body Part per Game	*Games*			*Practices*		
	Injury Type	*Percentage of Injuries*	*Injury per 1,000 Athlete-exposures*		*Percentage of Injuries*	*Injury per 1,000 Athlete-exposures*
Knee						
19.1%	Internal derangement	17.8	6.2	12%	12	0.5
	Contusion	1.3	0.46	–	–	–
Ankle						
15.6%	Ligament sprain	15.6	5.4	11.8%	11.8	0.5

% Injury Body Part per Game	Games			Practices		
	Injury Type	Percentage of Injuries	Injury per 1,000 Athlete-exposures		Percentage of Injuries	Injury per 1,000 Athlete-exposures
Shoulder 11.2%	Acromioclavicular joint injury	2.8	1	9.7%	1.8	0.1
	Ligament sprain	2.6	0.9		2.0	0.1
	Subluxation	2.1	0.7		2.4	0.1
	Contusion	1.9	0.7		1.4	0.1
	Muscle–tendon strain	1.8	0.6		2.1	0.1
Upper leg 7.3%	Contusion	3.7	1.3	12.6%	1.9	0.1
	Muscle–tendon strain	3.6	1.2		10.7	0.4
Head 6.8%	Concussion	6.8	2.3	5.5%	5.5	0.2
Pelvis/hip 3.7%	Muscle–tendon strain	1.9	0.6	5.2%	5.2	0.2
	Contusion	1.8	0.6		–	–
Lower leg 2.8%	Contusion	1.8	0.6	1%	1	0.04
	Fracture	1	0.3		–	–
Neck 1.8%	Nerve injury	1.8	0.6	1.5%	1.5	0.1
Ribs 1.4%	Contusion	1.4	0.5	0%	–	–
Lower back 1.2%	Muscle–tendon strain	1.2	0.4	2.7%	2.7	0.1
Patella 1.1%	Patella or patella tendon	1.1	0.4	1.6%	1.6	0.1
Foot 1.1%	Ligament sprain	1.1	0.4	1%	1	0.04
Hand 1%	Fracture	1	0.3	1%	1	0.04
Unspecified 1%	Unspecified	1	0.3	1.9%	1.9	0.1

Source: Data from Dick et al., 2007b.

competitive games and fall practices. The knee was the part of the body that was most commonly injured during a game (19.1% of all injuries), while the upper leg was the most common site of injury during practice (12.6% of all injuries). When injuries were reported as a body part group, the most common area was the lower extremity (54.7% and 50.8% in competitive games and practices, respectively) followed by the upper extremity (22.6% and 20.1% in games and practices, respectively), head/neck (11.5% and 10.1% in games and practices, respectively), and the trunk and back (9.9% and 13.2%, respectively). Approximately 1.4% and 5.9% of injuries occurring in both games and practices, respectively, were classified as "other" (Dick et al., 2007b).

Most injuries occur via direct contact with another player (see Figure 6.2). This is correct for both games and practice. Noncontact injuries were the second most frequent cause of injury in both games and practice sessions. Noncontact injuries generally occur from a player making a sharp cut and change in direction. The plant and twist of that move results in an ankle or knee injury, or possible muscle strain or tear from the sudden acceleration. The other major cause of injury was contact from a ball, ground, or other practice implements such as blocking sleds or blocking pads that may have resulted in missed time. There were also additional injuries that did not fit in any of the previously mentioned categories and simply were described as "other".

Subsequent research examining injury etiology reported similar findings regarding the mechanism of injury in football players (Kerr et al., 2016a). In the five-year assessment period, contact

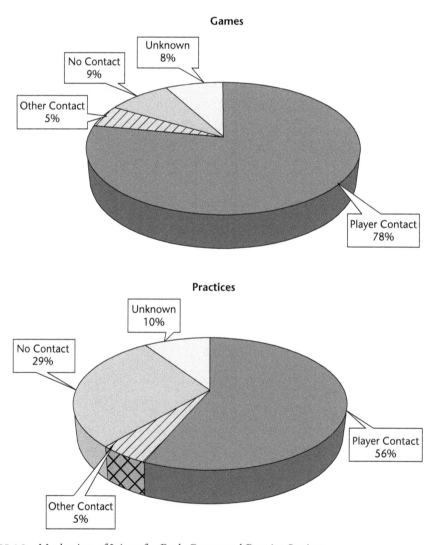

FIGURE 6.2   Mechanism of Injury for Both Games and Practice Sessions.

Source: Data from Dick et al., 2007b.

with another player accounted for 74.5% of total injuries during a game. This include injuries that resulted from tackling (20.4%), being tackled (20.6%), blocking (13.5%), being blocked (11.8%) or being stepped on, fell on, or kicked (7.7%). Noncontact injuries accounted for 14.3% of the injuries during a game, but accounted for 30.4% of the total injuries in practice sessions. Similar to the results of Dick and colleagues (2007b), the number of contact injuries during practices was also reduced (48.5%).

Running backs experienced the greatest percentage of injuries (19.6%) during a game. The second most frequently injured position was quarterback (17.5% of all injuries), followed by linebackers (15.5%), wide receivers (14.4%), defensive backs (11.7%), and defensive linemen (11.3%). Offensive linemen (9.9%) had the lowest frequency of injury (Dick et al., 2007b).

One study compared injury rates of high school and college football players (Shankar et al., 2007). A total of 100 high schools and 55 NCAA schools submitted 1,881 and 3,459 injury reports, respectively, via their online surveillance systems. Results indicated that the overall injury rate for the high school football player was 4.4 injuries per 1,000 athlete-exposures (12.0 and 2.6 for competition and practice sessions, respectively), while the injury rate for NCAA football players was 8.6 injuries per 1,000 player-exposures (40.2 and 5.8 for competition and practice sessions, respectively). Similar to previous reports, the risk for injury was significantly greater during games than practice sessions. The most frequent injury in the high school football player were ligament sprains (29% of the total injuries in practice and 33% in games), followed by muscle/tendon sprains (24% in practice and 10% in games) and contusions (13% in practice and 16% during games). Ligament sprains also accounted for the most frequent injury in college football players (25% of total injuries in practice sessions and 39% of total injuries in a game). Injuries to the lower body (hip, knee, ankle, and foot) accounted for 46.9% of the total injuries in the high school football player and 54.2% of the injuries in the NCAA football player. In contrast to what was previously reported in the college football player, the playing position that was most frequently injured in high school football was offensive linemen (17.9% of the total injuries) followed by running backs (15.5% of the injuries).

Positional comparison for injury rate needs to be put into appropriate context. In games, the quarterback is the second most frequently injured player (Dick et al., 2007b). But in practice sessions, the quarterback is often protected from any contact, and injury risk is minimized. To ensure that no one mistakes who the quarterback is during practice, he often wears a different color jersey. Injury risk for the other positions is likely a function of job responsibility. During each play, linemen have a specific blocking assignment, while skill position players often attempt to avoid contact. However, when the skill position player does make contact, the potential impact may be much greater than the linemen's, as impact occurs at a higher velocity of movement. However, linemen sustain a higher overall number of impacts, but skill position players had a greater incidence of severe impacts as reflected by a greater acceleration upon impact (Funk et al., 2012).

In 2004, the NCAA and high school injury collection information moved to a web-based platform, eliminating the need for athletic trainers to mail or fax their information to the NCAA. Using this new reporting format, Kerr and colleagues (2018) compared the injury rate in high school (2005–2016) and NCAA college (2004–2016) football players. An average of 100 high school football programs provided data to the high school surveillance program during the study period. An average of 43 NCAA member institutions (20 Division I, 7 Division II, and 16 Division III programs) participated during this study period. Results of this study indicated that the rate of injury in high school football was significantly lower than that seen in college football

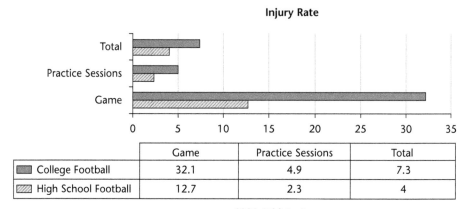

Injury Rate

	Game	Practice Sessions	Total
College Football	32.1	4.9	7.3
High School Football	12.7	2.3	4

1000 Athlete-Exposures

FIGURE 6.3   Injury Rate Comparisons Between High School and College Football.

Source: Data from Kerr et al., 2018.

TABLE 6.2 Injury Rate Comparisons Between NCAA Division I, Division II, and Division III Football Programs

NCAA Division		Athlete-Exposures	Injury Rate per 1,000 Athlete-Exposures
I	Game	1,552,554	4.6
	Practice	144,697	34.1
	Total	1,697,251	7.1[#]
II	Game	411,855	3.9
	Practice	38,338	29.6
	Total	450,193	6.1
III	Game	879,899	5.8
	Practice	94,134	30.2
	Total	974,032	8.1[*]

Source: Adapted from Kerr et al., 2018.

Notes: [#] = Significantly different than Division II; [*] = significantly different than Division I and Division II.

(see Figure 6.3). This was consistent across both games and practices. This is likely related to the greater strength and speed of the collegiate players that result in a greater impact at point of contact. In addition, the injury rate at Division NCAA III programs (combined for practice and games) was significantly greater than the injury rate observed at NCAA Division I and II programs, while the injury rate for Division I football programs (combined practice and games) was significantly greater than the injury rate observed at NCAA Division II programs (see Table 6.2).

Injury Rate Among NFL Players

The number of studies examining the injury rate in NFL players is very limited. Although there are a number of publications that have focused on return to play following various surgical procedures or treatments from a specific injury, the data regarding injury rate are limited. In 2015, Lawrence and colleagues reported on the incidence and patterns of all-cause injury and concussions in the NFL. The investigators examined the injury reports for each week for two competitive seasons (2012–2013 and 2013–2014 regular seasons for all 32 teams). Injury rates were reported as the number of injuries per 100 team games (TG) and injuries per 1,000 athletes at risk (AAR). An AAR is a participating athlete. There are 11 AARs per team at any time during a game. The denominator is calculated by multiplying the number of total games played by 11. Over the duration of the study, 984 games were evaluated, so 11 × 984 = 10,824 AAR. A total of 4,284 injuries were identified in 1,172 players during the two-year study duration. An injury occurred in 97.7% of the games played, while only 2.3% of the games were injury free. The all-cause injury rate was 435.37 per 100 TGs or 395.8 per 1,000 AARs. The injury rate per position can be seen in Figure 6.4. The position with the highest injury rate was defensive

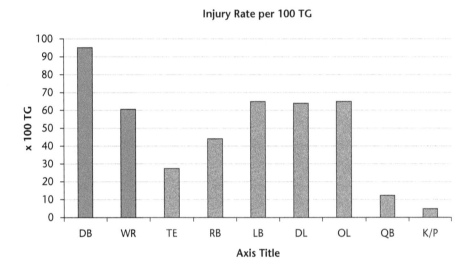

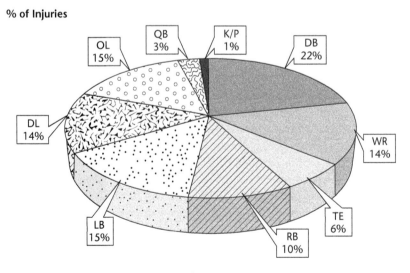

FIGURE 6.4   Injury Rate per Position in NFL Players.

DB = defensive backs; WR = wide receivers; TE = tight ends; RB = running backs; LB = linebackers; DL = defensive linemen; OL = offensive linemen; QB = quarterbacks; K/P = kickers and punters.

Source: Data from Lawrence et al., 2015.

backs, who accounted for 21.4% of all injuries. Linebackers and offensive linemen were the next most frequently injured positions (14.8% each). The lower extremity was the most frequent site of injury (61.9% of all injuries) in NFL players, followed by the upper extremity (18%), head and neck (10.2%), and finally the trunk (7.8%). Knees (17.8%) and ankles (12.4%) were the most common sites of injury in the lower extremity, while an injury to the shoulder (8.4% of total injuries) was the most common site in the upper extremity. Concussion (7.0%) and back (4.8%) accounted for the most injured site in the head and next, and trunk, respectively.

Lower extremity injuries appear to be the most common site of injury in football players. This is likely related to a number of factors that include sharp cuts, rapid accelerations that lead to noncontact injuries, and contact injuries that involve unprepared contact to lateral surface of joints. For instance, a lineman is knocked down and falls on the outside part of the knee of his teammate who is engaged with another opponent. In addition, the type of surface area that the athlete plays on may also impact injury risk. Hershman and colleagues (2012) compared injury rate of the lower extremity in NFL players playing on natural grass versus artificial grass surfaces. The investigators reported that playing on artificial surfaces resulted in a significantly greater risk for both ankle and knee injuries. Injury rates for ankle sprains and knee ligament sprains were 67% ($p < 0.001$) and 31% ($p < 0.001$) higher on artificial grass surfaces than on natural grass surfaces.

Effect of College Football Injury and NFL Career Performance

In Chapter 4 discussion was focused on the validity of performance assessments conducted at the NFL combine to predict future NFL performance. In addition to performance assessments, athletes invited to the combine also participate in a medical evaluation. All previous injuries and health histories are evaluated to determine the type of medical risk that a player presents. If a player is drafted and seriously hurt while practicing, which will result in him missing extensive time, he can be placed on the team's injured reserve list and his salary will be paid. This could be an expensive proposition if the player selected high in the draft is unable to play due to injury. Teams will attempt to get as much information to minimize the risk in a sport that already has a high risk for injury.

The only published study to have examined the effect of injures in college football players and their impact on NFL performance was published in 2017 (Beaulieu-Jones et al., 2017). In this study, the investigative team examined all college football players who participated in medical and performance testing at the NFL combine from 2009 to 2015. The players' medical records, imaging reports, physical examination findings, and self-reported medical history forms were examined. Performance variables included draft selection (e.g., round) and position-specific performance metrics for the player's first two NFL seasons. A total of 2,203 players were evaluated and 1,490 of those players were drafted (67.6%). An analysis of total collegiate games played revealed that players missed 2.7 ± 4.3 games during their collegiate career. Each player was reported to have sustained on average 3.8 ± 1.8 injuries during their college career. The effect on NFL draft status was interesting. Players drafted missed on average 2.5 ± 4.0 total games during their collegiate career, while players undrafted missed 3.3 ± 4.9 games. These differences were significant ($p < 0.001$). However, there was no significant difference in the number of injuries sustained during college among drafted players (3.9 ± 1.8) and undrafted players (3.8 ± 1.7). Thus, the severity of injury was more important, as interpreted by games missed, versus the number of injuries sustained.

The investigators also compared injury history to draft round by position. College injury history appeared to negatively affect draft position (e.g., round drafted in) for most football playing

TABLE 6.3 Effect of College Injury on NFL Position-Specific Performance

Position	Effect
Defensive backs	• Knee injuries appeared to result in significantly fewer tackles recorded • Hand injury resulted in fewer tackles recorded and fewer games played
Defensive linemen	• Knee injuries led to fewer games started, fewer mean tackles, fewer quarterback hits, and fewer mean sacks • Ankle injuries led to fewer games played, fewer games started, and fewer mean tackles
Linebackers	• Prior injury to the spine led to fewer games started and fewer overall tackles • Ankle injuries also led to fewer games started and fewer overall tackles
Offensive linemen	• Shoulder injuries led to fewer games played • Ankle injuries also led to fewer games played but interestingly also resulted in fewer penalty yards and fewer sacks allowed
Quarterbacks	• Shoulder injuries resulted in fewer games played during the first two years in the NFL (16.7 ± 9.9 games) compared to quarterbacks without prior shoulder injury (27 ± 7.4 games)
Running backs	• Most commonly sustained injuries in college involved the shoulder and ankle, but neither affected performance during the first two-years of their NFL career • Hand injuries led to fewer carries and fewer total yards.
Wide receivers	• Knee injuries led to fewer games started during the first two years in the NFL (7.2 ± 6.8) compared to running backs without prior knee injury (10.9 ± 10.1)
Tight ends	• Shoulder injuries led to fewer games played • Hand injuries led to fewer games played

Note: All results presented were significant (p < 0.05).

Source: Data adapted from Beaulieu-Jones et al., 2017.

positions. This was especially relevant for both offensive and defensive linemen. Defensive linemen with shoulder injuries were drafted significantly lower (draft position of 115.9 – mid-fourth round) than linemen who did not have a shoulder injury (draft position of 91.1 – end of third round), while offensive linemen with a shoulder injury demonstrated a similar significant effect (draft position of 122.9 mid-fourth round versus 96.1 – end of third round). The drop from late third round to fourth round was also noted in offensive linemen with a prior knee injury. Such a drop may have cost a previously injured player approximately $1 million in salary and bonus (see Chapter 4). The effect of specific injury patterns from college and how they subsequently impacted playing performance in the NFL are detailed in Table 6.3. The importance of this is that it can provide coaches and the front office personnel further information regarding potential performance effects in college players with a significant injury history. These results demonstrate that the best predictor of future performance, or injury, is to examine past history.

Injury Rate Among Youth Football Players

There is a scarcity of data examining injury risk in youth football. In one of the few studies to examine this issue, Caswell and colleagues (2016) examined a cohort of youth football players participating in a metropolitan youth football league for a two-year period (2011–2012). A total of 819 boys in the fifth to eighth grades participated in the league during the study period.

The average age of the children was 11.8 ± 1.2 years, and their football playing experience was 2.0 ± 1.8 years. The children played approximately eight games per season, which lasted nine weeks (one bye week). They also practiced twice per week. Injury data were collected by the league's athletic trainer. In total, 261 injuries were reported in 35,957 athlete-exposures for a total incident rate of 7.3 injuries per 1,000 athlete-exposures. Most injuries reported were minor (70.1%) that required no time loss. To keep this data in perspective, most other studies previously discussed would not label this as a reportable injury, and it would not count toward the injury rate. Only 29.9% of the injuries resulted in a removal and missing of a practice or game. The injury rate for these injuries was 2.2 per 1,000 athlete-exposures, which was much lower than that reported in all other leagues and reflects the level of speed and strength associated with youth football. A total of 4.9% of the youth players suffered a severe injury, which was defined as a fracture, sprain, strain, concussion, or eye injury.

Types of Injury

Tables 6.4 and 6.5 compare the injury location and type of injury for both high school and college football players in both competitive games and practice sessions, respectively. The most common area of injury in both practice and games for both high school and college football

TABLE 6.4 Comparison of Injury Location in High School and College Football Players

Body Part	High School Football				NCAA College Football			
	Game		Practice		Game		Practice	
	% of Injuries	Injury Rate/1,000 Athlete-Exposures	% of Injuries	Injury Rate/1,000 Athlete-Exposures	% of Injuries	Injury Rate/1,000 Athlete-Exposures	% of Injuries	Injury Rate/1,000 Athlete-Exposures
Lower Extremity	**42.8**		**43.7**		**56.5**		**55.4**	
• Hip/thigh/ upper leg	6.5	0.8	10.6	0.2	10.6	3.4	19.9	1.0
• Knee	16.5	2.1	13.3	0.3	20.2	6.5	15.3	0.7
• Lower leg	4.4	0.6	4.2	0.1	4.5	1.4	3.6	0.2
• Ankle	13.1	1.7	12.2	0.3	17.0	5.5	11.8	0.6
• Foot	2.3	0.3	3.4	0.1	4.2	1.4	4.8	0.2
Upper Extremity	**27.2**		**26.5**		**22.3**		**20.0**	
• Shoulder/ clavicle	13.1	1.7	10.9	0.3	13.2	4.2	12.1	0.6
• Arms/elbow	4.2	0.5	3.8	0.1	3.1	1.0	2.2	0.1
• Hand/wrist	9.9	1.3	11.8	0.3	6.0	1.9	5.7	0.3
Head and Neck	**24.1**		**20.0**		**13.9**		**12.3**	
• Head and face	21.2	2.7	17.0	0.4	10.0	3.2	9.3	0.5
• Neck	2.9	0.4	3.0	0.1	3.9	1.3	3.0	0.2
Trunk	**5.2**		**7.4**		**6.1**		**6.7**	
• Trunk	5.2	0.7	7.4	0.2	6.1	2.0	6.7	0.3

Source: Data from Kerr et al., 2018.

TABLE 6.5 Comparison of Types of Injury in High School and College Football Players

| Injury | High School Football | | | | NCAA College Football | | | |
| | Game | | Practice | | Game | | Practice | |
	% of Injuries	Injury Rate/1,000 Athlete-Exposures	% of Injuries	Injury Rate/1,000 Athlete-Exposures	% of Injuries	Injury Rate/1,000 Athlete-Exposures	% of Injuries	Injury Rate/1,000 Athlete-Exposures
Concussion	20.4	0.4	15.8	2.6	9.4	0.4	8.4	3.0
Contusion	14.9	0.2	10.9	1.9	15.4	0.5	10.0	4.9
Dislocation	5.1	0.1	4.1	0.6	2.0	0.1	1.9	0.6
Fracture/ avulsion	11.7	0.3	11.1	1.5	6.2	0.2	3.9	2.0
Laceration	0.7	0.01	0.6	0.1	0.4	0.03	0.5	0.1
Ligament sprain	29.0	0.5	24.2	3.7	38.9	1.2	26.0	12.5
Muscle/ tendon strain	9.1	0.4	18.1	1.2	12.6	1.2	25.4	4.0
Other	9.1	0.3	15.2	1.2	15.2	1.1	23.9	4.9

Source: Data from Kerr et al., 2018.

players was the lower extremity. Injuries to the lower extremity though were approximately 12–14% greater in the college player. This may be related to the greater size and speed of the college athlete. The most commonly injured body part in both practices and games was the head/face for the high school athlete (21.2% and 17.0%, respectively), but for the college football player the most commonly injured body part was the knee (20.2%) in games and the hip/thigh/upper leg during practices (19.9%). The most common type of injury during games were ligament sprains for both high school (29.0%) and college (38.9%) football players. Ligament sprains were also the most common injury in practice for both levels of players. Although the incident of concussions during a game for the high school football player was slightly more than twice than seen in the college athletes (20.4% versus 9.4%, respectively), the relative rate of injury per 1,000 athlete-exposures was the same (0.4 per 1,000 athlete-exposures) between the different levels of football.

Concussion

Concussions have been around the game of football since its inception. The number of deaths occurring on the football field at the turn of the twentieth century nearly led President Theodore Roosevelt to ban the game (Klein et al., 2012). Although "getting your skull smashed in" wasn't the only danger, the rule changes and the inclusion of helmets into the game was designed to reduce the risk of head injuries. However, helmets didn't become mandatory until 1943 (Stamp, 2012). According to Stamp (2012), the first use of a helmet may have occurred in the Army–Navy game of 1893 by Joseph Mason Reeve, who had been hit in the head so often that his doctor indicated that the next hit could result in "instant insanity". Mr. Reeve later became Admiral Reeve and is known as the *Father of Carrier Aviation*. Mr. Reeve went to his shoemaker to design some form of leather protection for his head and the concept of the leather helmet was born. Although the use of leather helmets continued into the 1950s, the first production of a plastic helmet was presented by John T. Riddel in 1939, but the advent of World War II and the demand for plastic put this invention on hold. It wasn't until the end of the war that the plastic helmet was reintroduced. Still, facemasks did not appear until the 1950s and padding and the use of a chin strap added during the same time period increased the safety. The helmet has continued to evolve today to maximize player safety.

In the past 20 years, there have been additional efforts focused on concussion recognition, prevention, and stricter guidelines defined to regulate safe return to play. To help reduce occurrence, it becomes important to determine how they occur. Concussions generally occur for the defensive player (e.g., defensive linemen, linebackers, and defensive backs) when they tackle a ball carrier, while the act of getting tackled is the primary mechanism for offensive players, except offensive linemen who are most often concussed in the act of blocking an opponent (Kerr et al., 2018). Changes in rules, such as the targeting rule, which was enacted in 2010, were designed to help reduce the risk of concussion. In the injury surveillance study that examined college football injuries between 1988 and 2004, concussions accounted for 6.8% of the injuries during competition (2.34 injury rate per 1,000 athlete-exposures) and 5.5% of the injuries in practice (0.21 injury rate per 1,000 athlete-exposures) (Dick et al., 2007b). Ten years later, and three years after the rule change, concussions accounted for 9.4% of the injuries during competition (3.01 injury rate per 1,000 athlete-exposures) and 8.4% of the injuries sustained during practice (0.4 injury rate per 1,000 athlete-exposures). During the same time frame, the rate of concussions also elevated from 2.6 per 1,000 athlete-exposures to 3.5 per 1,000 athlete-exposures. This increase, however, may be more of a function of education and recognition than anything else (Westermann et al., 2016). The rule change has also been suggested to increase the number of lower extremity injuries, as lower extremity injury increased from 20.5 per 1,000 athlete-exposures in 2009 to 23.6 per 1,000 athlete-exposures in 2015.

Etiology of Concussion Injury and Its Physiological Effect

Injuries to the head are not the most common injuries in football at any level (Dick et al., 2007b; Kerr et al., 2018); however, injuries to the head may have the greatest long-term health consequences. Concussion is a form of brain injury that is on the mild or less severe side of the brain injury spectrum. It is considered to be a mild traumatic brain injury (mTBI) that is generally self-limited in duration and resolution (Harmon et al., 2013). Concussions in football occur when a force (e.g., helmet, forearm, shoulder, or leg) makes appreciable contact directly at the head or indirectly by contact elsewhere that forces the head to move linearly or rotationally (e.g., such as during a whiplash injury) at a sufficient force that is transmitted to the brain (Harmon et al., 2013). The resulting forces, either direct or indirect, cause brain tissue to forcefully contact the skull. A cascade of events is initiated that includes a disruption of the neuronal cell membranes, damage to the blood–brain barrier (BBB), and axonal shearing (Barkhoudarian et al., 2016; Chen et al., 2019; Giza and Hovda, 2014). This results in an overload of tightly regulated ion channels causing the widespread release of various neurotransmitters and excitatory amino acids such as glutamate (Barkhoudarian et al., 2016). The resulting ionic imbalance leads to excitotoxicity, inflammation, and apoptosis (Chen et al., 2019; Giza and Hovda, 2014). The Na/K ATPase pump is activated to restore ionic balance in the brain depleting energy stores. Depletion of energy stores is also the result of decreased cerebral blood flow and mitochondrial function due to the initial damage (Barkhoudarian et al., 2016). The cell processes needed to reestablish ionic equilibrium deplete energy stores and increase metabolic stress, leading to necrosis (Chen et al., 2019). These changes are thought to be self-limiting and transient, but it may result in more lasting pathophysiological changes or permanent damage during repeat injury (Barkhoudarian et al., 2016; Chen et al., 2019). Excessive physical activity or cognitive overload prior to complete recovery may prolong neurodysfunction (Harmon et al., 2013), and this may be of greater concern in the young athlete (Shrey et al., 2011).

Symptoms Associated With Concussions

There are a number of signs and symptoms associated with a concussion. A headache is the most common symptom, with dizziness being the second most common symptom (Kerr et al., 2016b; O'Connor et al., 2017). Loss of consciousness is also a risk but occurs in only 4% of the occurrences of a concussion (Kerr et al., 2016b). The complete list of symptoms associated with concussions experienced by players in youth, high school, and college football players are listed in Table 6.6. Kerr and colleagues (2016b) examined concussion occurrence and symptoms in youth, high school, and college football players over three seasons (2012–2014). In players concussed, the average number of symptoms per occurrence was about 5.5 ± 3.1. Although symptom resolution is often observed within seven days post-injury (Harmon et al., 2013), this may not represent a complete cognitive recovery. Neuropsychological impairments may still persist. Specific symptoms may provide some indication of recovery time. Harmon and colleagues (2013) indicated that dizziness at the time of injury may be a predictor of a recovery that will take longer than 21 days. In addition, the presence of three or more symptoms at the time of injury is often associated with a longer recovery.

TABLE 6.6 Concussion-Related Symptoms in Youth, High School, and College Football Players

Symptom	Symptoms Reported by Athletes with Concussion (%)			
	Youth (n = 177)	High School (n = 825)	College (n = 410)	Total (n = 1,412)
Dizziness	79.7	76.7	69.5	75.0
Headache	98.9	95.0	90.7	94.3
Nausea/vomiting	35.6	34.5	26.3	32.3
Tinnitus	14.7	10.3	6.1	9.6
Loss of balance	32.8	34.5	45.1	37.4
Visual disturbance	20.9	22.9	32.4	25.4
Sensitivity to light	31.6	49.6	50.7	47.7
Sensitivity to noise	19.8	39.4	31.7	34.7
Posttraumatic amnesia	10.2	12.6	14.9	13.0
Retrograde amnesia	3.4	8.4	12.7	9.0
Difficulty concentrating	54.2	62.1	60.0	60.5
Disorientation	35.6	27.5	41.2	32.5
Loss of consciousness	1.7	3.6	4.9	3.8
Excess drowsiness	23.2	36.1	27.3	31.9
Excess excitability	4.0	6.9	4.1	5.7
Excess irritability	8.5	17.5	13.2	15.1
Insomnia	1.7	22.7	24.6	20.6

Source: Data from Kerr et al., 2016b.

Epidemiology

One of the initial examinations focusing on the epidemiology of concussions was published by Dr. Kevin Guskiewicz and his colleagues at the University of North Carolina (Guskiewicz et al., 2000). His investigation focused on the incidence of concussion in both high school and collegiate football players, the symptoms associated with concussion and return to play. Of the 17,549 football players investigated, 888 sustained at least one concussion (5.1%). Of these players, 131 (14.7%) sustained a second concussion during the same season. The investigative team noted that players who sustained one concussion during the season were three times more likely to sustain a second concussion during the same season than those players who had not sustained a previous injury.

In a subsequent study, the concussion risk of youth, high school, and college football players were examined in more than 20,300 athlete-seasons (4,092 youth, 11,957 high school, and 4,305 college) in athletes ranging in age from 5 to 23 (Dompier et al., 2015). A total of 1,198 concussions were reported in the two-year study. The number of concussions reported in youth football players was 141 (11.8%), 795 in high school football players (66.4%) and 262 in college football players (21.9%). Concussions comprised 9.6%, 4.0%, and 8.0% of all injuries reported in the injury surveillance programs used by each of these organizations. This represented a risk level of 2.4, 2.0, and 3.7 per 1,000 athlete-exposures for youth, high school, and college athletes, respectively, during competition. The risk of concussion during practice was 0.6, 0.7, and 0.5 per 1,000 athlete-exposures for youth, high school, and college athletes, respectively. Clearly, the risk for concussion was much higher during competition than practice.

In 2017, O'Connor and colleagues (2017) examined high school athletes for three years (2011–2014). They used the National Athletic Treatment, Injury and Outcomes Network (NATION) surveillance program, which provided a convenience sample of 147 high schools drawn from 26 states to compile data on 31 sports. As expected, the sport with the highest incidence of concussion was football. However, the relative rate of concussive injury was the highest recorded in any other study. They reported a concussion injury risk of 9.2 per 1,000 athlete-exposures. This was nearly three times greater than any previous report. Similar to other studies, the rate of injury was far greater in competition than practice (19.9 versus 6.8 per 1,000 athlete-exposures, respectively). Part of this issue may very well be related to the lack of a universal agreement on the definition of a concussion (Guskiewicz et al., 2003).

In the past 15+ years, there have been several studies conducted on the epidemiology of concussions in NFL players (Casson et al., 2010; Clark et al., 2017; Pellman et al., 2004). Casson and colleagues (2010) examined the effect of various rule changes on two separate six-year periods of play (1996–2001 and 2002–2007). Average concussions per season in the first six years was 147.8 concussions (4.8 concussion per team), which was reduced to 3.7% in the second six-year period (142.3 concussion per year and 4.4 concussions per team). Quarterbacks, wide receivers, and tight ends were the most vulnerable positions for concussion. The concussion rate for NFL games during a 19-year period (1996–2014) can be observed in Table 6.7. No differences were noted between the 1996–2007 competitive seasons. However, the rate between 2010 and 2014 was significantly greater than the first two reporting periods (Clark et al., 2017). As discussed earlier, this is likely a function of education and heightened sensitivity to the injury compared to previous years.

Clark and colleagues (2017) examined several risk factors associated with the game and how they impacted concussion risk in the NFL. As might be expected, a greater number of concussions occurred in the second half of a game, when the player was fatigued. Although the investigators hypothesized that closing distance and anticipation would be related to concussion, they

TABLE 6.7 Concussion Rate per Game in the NFL – Study Comparison

Study	Period	Total Number of Concussions	Total Number of Games	Concussion Rate per Game
Pellman et al., 2004	1996–2001	787	1,913	0.41
Casson et al., 2010	2002–2007	758	1,995	0.38
Clark et al., 2017	2010–2014	871	1,324	0.66*

Source: Adapted from Clark et al., 2017.

in fact were not. Most concussive hits occurred at a distance less than 10 yards, and players were more apt to be concussed even if they anticipated the contact.

Risk of Reinjury

One of the bigger concerns associated with a concussion is the athlete's return to play prior to being fully recovered. A concussive event results in a cascade of ionic, metabolic, and physiological changes that effect cerebral function for days or weeks. It is important to appreciate the impact of a football game and the physiological changes resulting from these impacts, even when a concussive event is not recorded. In a study examining football players following at least two months of competing, investigators using dynamic contrast-enhanced magnetic resonance imaging reported significantly greater BBB permeability in both gray and white matter of the cerebral cortex, with focal BBB lesions located in the base of temporal, frontal, parietal, and occipital lobes (Weissberg et al., 2014). These lesions were found without any difference in *Sideline Concussion Assessment Tools* and *Standardized Assessment of Concussion Scores* between the players and the nonplaying control group. These results demonstrate the potential disruption of the BBB from sub-concussive events that may lower the threshold for a concussive event or highlight the risk for an error in an expedited return to play.

In a study examining the acute effects and recovery time following concussion in college football players, McCrea and colleagues (2003) examined 1,631 college football players in 15 NCAA institutions over three seasons (1999–2001). Of these athletes, 94 were diagnosed with concussion. A cohort of 56 athletes, who were uninjured, were used as a control group. These control athletes were selected from the teams of the concussed athletes. Concussed athletes and control athletes completed several assessments to examine post-concussive symptoms, cognitive functioning, and postural stability. The results of these assessments are depicted in Figure 6.5. The test battery consisted of the *Graded Symptom Checklist*, which examines post-concussive symptoms, and the *Standardized Assessment of Concussion*, which measures cognitive function, including memory, orientation, and neurological screening. In addition, the battery included the *Balance Error Scoring System*, which measures postural stability, and the *Neuropsychological Test Battery*, which also assesses cognitive function, attention, anterograde memory, processing speed, and mental flexibility. Loss of consciousness was experienced by 6.4% of the concussed athletes (mean duration was 30 s), post-traumatic amnesia was experienced by 19.1% of the concussed athletes (mean duration of 90 min), and retrograde amnesia was experienced by 7.4% of the concussed athletes (mean duration was 120 min). No loss of consciousness or amnesia was experienced by 77.8% of the athletes concussed. Acute symptoms were clear following the concussive event and postgame/practice assessments. Differences were seen through day 5 of recovery, but most symptoms returned to baseline by day 7.

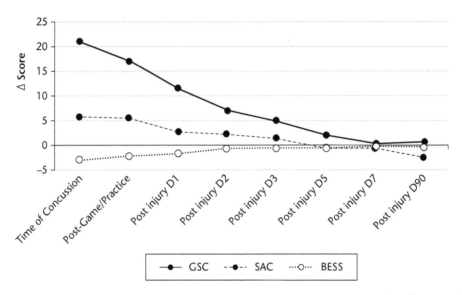

FIGURE 6.5 Post-Concussion Recovery Pattern Comparisons Between Concussed College Football
Players and Controls.

GSC = graded symptom checklist; SAC = standard assessment of concussion; BESS = balance error scoring system.
Source: Data adapted from McCrea et al., 2003.

Cognitive impairment was most severe immediately after injury, stayed impaired through
day 5, but appeared to be resolved by day 7. Balance deficits were most severe immediately
following concussion but appeared to resolve by day 5 post-injury. The results of this study
clearly demonstrated the need for a seven-day recovery period from mild concussive injury.
What is most concerning is the return to play also comes with an inherent risk for future
injury. Guskiewicz and colleagues (2003) reported that a previous concussive event increases
the risk for future concussion threefold. In addition, an increase in the number of concussions
was associated with a longer duration of symptom resolution in subsequent concussions. In
addition, loss of consciousness was associated with a greater resolution of symptoms, and any
amnesia associated with the concussive event trended toward a greater duration of time before
resolution of symptoms (Guskiewicz et al., 2003).

Blood Markers for Brain Injury During a Football Season

There have been several investigations that have examined changes in biomarkers to provide
some indication of neurodysfunction or concussion following a game (Rogatzki et al., 2016)
or throughout a competitive football season (Marchi et al., 2013; Oliver et al., 2017, 2019;
Rogatzki et al., 2018). In a single acute study, examining the effect of a football game on select
biomarkers of brain injury, blood was obtained from 17 NCAA Division III football players
two days before and 1 h following a competitive game. Serum was analyzed for neuronal specific enolase (NSE) and protein S100B. S100B is thought to be an indicator of BBB disruption
(Marchi et al., 2004). Although both markers are used to measure brain damage, none of the
players participating in the study suffered a head injury or concussion. Regardless, significant elevations were noted in both NSE and S100B, following the game NSE concentrations

increased from 7.0 µg·L^{-1} before the game to 13.1 µg·L^{-1} postgame. Similarly, S100B concentrations increased from 0.013 to 0.069 µg·L^{-1} postgame. Most importantly, these biomarkers remained within normal physiological levels and the increase observed at postgame may reflect possible muscle damage or normal fluid volume shifts that caused changes in these biomarker concentrations.

Changes in S100B were also examined during a season of competition. Marchi and colleagues (2013) appear to have been the first investigative team to examine changes in S100B in competitive football players. They examined three college football teams. A total of 57 players volunteered for this study. Blood was obtained in 30 of these players 24 h before the game, 1 h and 24 h postgame. Twenty-seven players gave blood samples at baseline (prior to any football-related activity), 24 h before the game and 1 h following five consecutive home games. Complete season data were available for only 15 players. No differences were noted in S100B concentrations in players with previous history of concussion compared to players without any previous history, and no differences were noted between playing positions. The investigators noted that elevations in postgame S100B concentrations returned relatively quickly to baseline levels, and that baseline levels remained consistent throughout the season suggesting that a single preseason measure may suffice to examine changes in biological biomarkers during a season of competition. Baseline and pregame S100B concentrations were below the threshold indicative of a BBB disruption. However, nine players experienced a postgame elevation above the BBB disruption threshold, and only five players displayed this disruption on more than two occasions. One of the most interesting findings from this study involved the significant correlation between the number and severity of head hits and the change in S100B (r^2 = 0.51). These results were supported in a subsequent study on NCAA Division III football players (Rogatzki et al., 2016).

Changes in tau protein, a marker for axonal damage in the brain, were measured in football players during the course of a NCAA Division I season (Oliver et al., 2017). The microtubule cytoskeleton plays a fundamental role in establishing and maintaining the integrity of axons and dendrites, and tau protein is responsible in part for stabilizing these microtubules (Scott et al., 1992). The presence of tau in the circulation may be indicative of a loss of integrity and stabilization of the microtubules, resulting in the development of neurofibrillary tangles, a pathological characteristic of chronic traumatic encephalopathy (CTE) (McKee et al., 2013), which will be discussed in much greater detail in Chapter 7. In the study, eight resting blood samples were obtained: at the start of summer conditioning, end of summer conditioning and prior to the start of preseason training camp, end of preseason training camp, and then five times during the course of the season. All inseason measurements occurred on a Monday morning following a Saturday game. No more than 28 days lapsed between inseason measures. No differences from baseline were noted in tau concentrations during the competitive season, except for a decrease at the end of summer training camp. Comparisons between starters and nonstarters revealed that starters had a higher mean tau concentration at baseline and at two inseason measuring points toward the end of the season compared to nonstarters. Calculation of tau area under the curve (AUC) over the duration of the season resulted in a significantly higher value in starters than nonstarters (see Figure 6.6).

In a follow-up study, Oliver and colleagues (2019) examined tau protein and neurofilament light polypeptide (NF-L) in NCAA college football players during a season of competition. NF-L is also a biomarker of head trauma that is primarily found in axons. NF-L functions to provide structural support to the neuron, together with tau protein, their measurement provides a degree of understanding regarding axonal cytoskeleton integrity and stability (Siedler et al., 2014). The sampling times were similar to the previous study, with the exception that there was

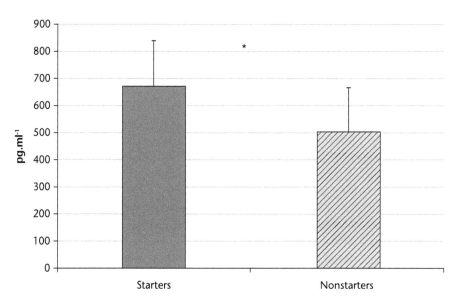

FIGURE 6.6 AUC Tau Protein Comparisons Between Starters and Nonstarters in a NCAA Division I Football Season. ★ = significant difference between groups.

Source: Data from Oliver et al., 2017.

no blood measurement during the summer conditioning session. Results of the AUC analysis of plasma concentrations of tau protein revealed a significantly lower ($p = 0.05$) response in starters (417 ± 129 pg·ml^{-1} day) than in nonstarters (521 ± 163 pg·ml^{-1} day) during the season. No changes were noted during the season in either starters or nonstarters. Elevations in NF-L were noted from pre- to post-preseason training camp in both starters and nonstarters. However, the increases in nonstarters were not significant, and changes in serum NF-L during the season did not differ from baseline levels throughout the season. In contrast, NF-L concentrations in starters were significantly elevated by the end of preseason training camp and remained elevated throughout the seasons. The higher serum concentrations of NF-L observed in starters resulted in a significantly greater AUC for that group compared to nonstarters ($1,605 \pm 655$ pg·ml^{-1} day versus $1,067 \pm 272$ pg·ml^{-1} day, respectively; $p = 0.007$).

The difference in results regarding the change in tau protein concentrations between the two studies by Oliver and colleagues (2017, 2019) are difficult to explain. It is possible that tau protein is not a consistent marker for sub-concussive blows to the head, or perhaps differences in data collection points may have had a greater effect. Blood collections during the initial study occurred on a Monday morning following a Saturday game (~40 h). However, in the latter study, blood collection varied from 36 to 72 h following the game. Considering that tau concentrations return to baseline fairly quickly, this may potentially explain the contrasting results. Although elevations in circulating concentrations of tau protein have been reported to persist for 72 h after injury (Gill et al., 2017), this generally occurs following a concussive event. Interestingly, changes in serum concentrations of NF-L may be more sensitive to the repeated head trauma during a season of competition.

To date, there is no widespread acceptance of a specific biomarker that can be used to determine or predict a sub-concussive brain injury. There has been a recent attempt to examine genetic biomarkers that may potentially predict a player's risk for concussion or post-concussion recovery and outcome. Terrell and colleagues (2018) examined 1,056 college athletes over a 9+ year period. In total, 133 concussions were recorded (12.1% occurrence rate). A number of potential genetic biomarkers were examined. The investigators reported a significant positive association between interleukin 6-receptor (IL-6R) CC genotype (SNP rs22281450) and increased concussion risk (p = 0.001). In addition, the APOE4 allele was associated with a reduced risk of concussion (p = 0.03). Associations between concussion and the remaining polymorphisms were not significant. Unadjusted and adjusted logistic regression analyses showed a significant association between IL-6R CC and concussion [(odds ratio) OR 3.48; 95% CI 1.58–7.65; p = 0.002] and between the APOE4 allele and concussion (OR 0.61; 95% CI 0.38–0.96; p = 0.04). Although results were interesting, more research is needed to provide further validity to these results. Furthermore, these genetic markers have also been suggested to be associated with a number of other neuropathological conditions such as Alzheimer's disease, Parkinson's disease, and multiple sclerosis (Rothaug et al., 2016). Whether there is an ethical issue with such testing still has yet to be debated.

Return to Play Protocols

The decision to return to play is an important one for both the player and the medical staff. The player may physically feel fine, and/or he feels the pressure of playing in an important game exerted by himself or by his teammates or coaches. A wrong decision can have significant impact on his long-term health. This is the reason that set protocols have been developed to help the medical staff, both team physician and athletic trainer make the right decision regarding the long-term health of the athlete. There is a specific graduated return to play protocol that has been recommended (Harmon et al., 2013). It is designed to gradually move the player from complete recovery to light activity to eventually contact drills to help him regain confidence and ensure that he returns as healthy as possible.

Kerr and colleagues (2016b) examined the return to play in youth, high school, and college football players who were concussed. Return-to-play time varied by the level of competition. A return-to-play exceeding 30 days was seen in 19.5% of the high school football players who were concussed, which was greater than either youth (16.3%) or college players (7.0%). Across all levels of play, 15.5% of the players concussed will miss at least 30 days of football. In general, 37.8% of the concussed athletes across all levels of competition will return to play within 7–13 days, while 26.3% will return between 15 and 19 days.

Kumar and colleagues (2014) were interested in examining short-term return to play protocols in NFL players. They hypothesized that on-field performance would be different in players who return to play within seven days post-concussion compared with players who missed at least one game due to concussion. A total of 124 players who sustained 131 concussions qualified for this study. Seventy-two (55%) of the players who were concussed did not miss a game due to the concussion, while 59 of the players (45%) missed at least one game. Interestingly, players who missed at least one game were younger (26.0 versus 27.2 years, p = 0.037) and less experienced (4.1 versus 5.3 years of NFL experience; p = 0.025) and played in less career games (44.3 versus 64.1 games; p = 0.004) at the time of injury. No other differences were noted. No significant difference was noted in objective measures of football playing performance from pre to post-injury in either group, suggesting that not missing a game did not negatively impact football playing performance. This resulted in the investigators not accepting their hypothesis. They suggested that the more experienced players may have known how to mask or not report their symptoms to expedite a faster return to the field. In addition, the more later in the season that the concussion had occurred, the greater the chance that no games would be missed. This is likely related to the greater importance of games later on in the season. Further, the investigators suggested that the younger players may have been exposed to a more conservative concussion protocol guidelines during high school and college and may have been more willing to report their post-concussive symptoms.

Summary

This chapter provided an overview of the injury risk associated with playing the game of football across a spectrum of various levels of competition. In addition, the type of injury and location of injury was compared across the various levels of play. Specific focus and attention was given to concussion injury. Injury patterns and recovery aspects from specific injuries such as ACL sprains, shoulder dislocations, etc. were beyond the scope of this book. Readers interested in specific return-to-play guidelines for injuries common to football are directed to the sport medicine literature. There have also been several efforts in the world of sport science to explore various assessments to predict risk for injury. Considering that there is little to no universal agreement or acceptance regarding such assessments, it was decided not to focus on that topic for this chapter.

7

MEDICAL ISSUES ASSOCIATED WITH RETIRED PLAYERS

Introduction

In 1984, a book titled *Death in the Locker Room* by Dr. Bob Goldman and colleagues was published. In the book, they detailed a survey that he was alleged to have given to 198 world-class athletes. These athletes were asked: If you could take a pill that would guarantee you winning every competition you would enter for the next five years, from the Olympic decathlon to Mr. Universe, but would have one major drawback: it would kill you five years after you took it. Would you still take the pill? He reported that more than 103 or 52% of the athletes surveyed indicated that they would still take the pill. Even though it was illegal and would kill them, the athletes still believed that it was worth the sacrifice. Whether this survey was real or not may not be important. It was never published in a peer-reviewed scientific journal, and later studies failed to support these numbers (Connor et al., 2013; Hoffman et al., 2008a). However, his story highlighted the mindset of many elite athletes whose aspirations were to achieve the ultimate in athletic experiences.

In the 1970s through 1990s, many football players dreaming of playing or who were already playing in the National Football League (NFL) decided to use anabolic steroids to enhance their chances of playing or remaining in the league. At the time it was not illegal, there was no testing, and it was also quite commonly used. Anecdotally, reports have suggested that 40–90% of the players in the league were using anabolic steroids in the 1970s and 1980s, it was more prevalent among the linemen (Johnson, 1985). Unfortunately, there is very limited scientific evidence regarding the extent of its use. The Sports Illustrated article may have been the closest explanation of what it was like for NFL players. In an attempt to examine the issue of anabolic steroid use and potential injury, Horn and colleagues (2009) surveyed 2,411 former NFL players, who participated between the 1940s and 1990s. Their results indicated that 9.1% of the former players self-admitted to using androgens, but numbers increased to 20.3% of the athletes who played during the 1980s. However, those numbers are quite low and should be interpreted with appropriate context. In the 1980s, there were 28 teams with approximately 90–100 players per team per year going to training camp. This would equate to a rough estimate of 28,000 player-years. A total of 518 athletes who played in the 1980s completed the questionnaire. Although the study by Horn et al. (2009) was the first serious attempt to scientifically examine androgen use patterns in former NFL players, many players were likely very reluctant to speak with investigators regarding anabolic steroid use in an era of high scrutiny that occurred following the Congressional hearings of anabolic steroid use among professional baseball players.

The use of anabolic steroids among players in the NFL has led to limited discussion or information on the risks or possibly benefits to the athlete's long-term health. In general, there is limited information regarding the use of androgens and long-term health of athletes (Hoffman et al., 2009c). There is some evidence suggesting that androgen use in NFL athletes was associated with greater risk for back pain, osteoarthritis, depression, and attention-deficit disorder during their retirement from professional football (Horn et al., 2009). However, the use of anabolic steroids was also associated with a reduced risk of diabetes and cancer (Horn et al., 2009). Although the issue of mortality was not examined, others examining European bodybuilders reported a greater risk for early mortality in individuals with a known history of androgen use (Petersson et al., 2006). Differences in androgen administration (dose and frequency) between strength/power athletes such as football players and bodybuilders are quite different (Hoffman et al., 2009c), and the risks associated with these different use patterns would likely differ as well. Interestingly, there is evidence to support neuroprotective effects of androgens (Nguyen et al., 2010), as well as potential neural dysfunction when used in pharmacological dosages (Selakovic et al., 2017). Considering the amount of funding that has gone into the study of concussion, it is surprising that little to no effort has been spent examining the potential effects of androgen use during the athlete's career and long-term health.

The issue of concussion and brain health has been in the media for quite some time. The movie "Concussion" starring Will Smith put the issue of chronic traumatic encephalopathy (CTE) on the forefront of all sports media for a while in 2015. The movie was based on the exposé "Game Brain" by Jeanne Marie Laskas, published in 2009 by GQ magazine. The movie was set in 2002 and provided a picture of the issues that were faced by many former NFL players. However, it is not the only issue facing retired athletes. Orthopedic problems, including arthritis, cardiovascular health, and metabolic syndrome, and neurological health, including depression and cognitive function, are all issues that have been raised in the retired football player. These issues are the focus of this chapter.

Do Former Football Players Age Well?

In 2004, 36 of the 41 members of the 1969 New York Jets Super Bowl Championship team were contacted by the former team physicians (Nicholas et al., 2007). The Super Bowl roster had 40 players, as one player was inactive due to injury. Three of the players were deceased at the time of the survey, and two players could not be contacted. The investigators were interested in examining how these men compared to age-matched peers. Players completed two questionnaires: an SF-36 health survey and a health- and football-specific questionnaire. The SF-36 questionnaire is composed of 36 separate questions relating to physical and mental health. The average age of the retired football players was 62 ± 3 years (range: 58–75 years). In 1969, one of the players was diagnosed with hypertensive and 20 players had significant orthopedic problems that required surgery and/or prolonged treatment. The NFL career of the players in the study averaged 8.3 ± 3.8 years. Of the 36 players surveyed, 23 retired voluntarily, 8 were cut and not picked up by another team, and 5 were forced to retire because of injury. When asked if their playing careers were fulfilling, 94% of the players answered somewhat fulfilling to very fulfilling. Interestingly, when players were asked, "In retrospect, if you had known what you know now, would you still have chosen to play professional football?", 34 replied they would still play and 2 said they would not. After 35 years, the most common medical issue was arthritis (67%) – the knee was the most predominant site in 71% of the players with arthritis. Other common medical issues reported were hypertension (54%) and chronic back pain (54%), while the remaining issues were limited to less than 14% (e.g., heart disease, cancer, stroke, kidney disease) of the former players. Five players (14%) had no medical issues and 20 players (56%) had more than one concurrent medical issue. SF-36 scores for physical and mental health for the retired football players were not different from age-matched norms. The results of the study indicated that aging in former NFL players caused no greater health issues than of other aging adults. In addition, despite the physical stress associated with the game of football, and the significant orthopedic issues experienced by these players, the risk of arthritis during their retirement was no different than their age-matched peers (Nicholas et al., 2007).

In 2012, the mortality rate of a cohort of 3,439 NFL players identified by a pension fund database of vested players with at least five credited playing seasons between 1959 and 1988 were compared through 2007 to the US population of men stratified by age and race (Baron et al., 2012; Lehman et al., 2012). The cohort was followed for 27 ± 9 years after retirement from the NFL, and the median age for players who were still alive at the study's end date was 57 years. Compared to the general US population, the former player's overall mortality and mortality from cancer and cardiovascular disease (CVD) were significantly lower than age-matched controls (Baron et al., 2012). An interesting observation was made regarding position comparisons and CVD. Defensive linemen had a 42% higher CVD mortality compared to the US population of men, whereas offensive linemen had no increase (Baron et al., 2012). Further, the examination of neurodysfunction yielded very interesting and concerning results. The neurodegenerative mortality was three times higher than that of the general American population, and four times higher for Alzheimer's disease and amyotrophic lateral sclerosis (Lehman et al., 2012).

In a follow-up study examining causes of death in former NFL players, a cohort of 9,778 former NFL players with at least one year in the NFL, whose last season was between 1986 and 2012, was examined (Lincoln et al., 2018). The median age of those alive at data analysis was 41 years (range: 24–68 years), whereas the median age at death was 38 years (range: 23–61 years). Two percent of players examined were deceased, with the most common cause of death being CVD (21%), violence (17%), and car accidents (15%). Violence and car accidents were the most common reason for death before the age of 35, and in particularly among nonwhites. Deaths from CVD and cancer were more prevalent among those aged 35–54. The standardized mortality ratio (SMR) was calculated from the ratio of observed to expected number of deaths. In comparison to the American population, former NFL players had a significantly lower overall mortality rate (see Table 7.1). Overall mortality was significantly lower than the general population across race, football playing position, and years in the NFL. In addition, mortality from CVD was significantly lower for both Caucasian and African American players compared to their general population peers.

The BMI is used as index to determine obesity and is commonly used among family physicians to provide a risk assessment of health. Many clinicians examining NFL players have described the increase in BMI among players over the last 40 years. The BMI of the 1969 Super Bowl champion New York Jets was 28.7 ± 3.0 (Nicholas et al., 2007). The BMI of the 2012 Super Bowl champion New York Giants was 32.5 (Pryor et al., 2014), indicating an increase in obesity for NFL champions over 43 years. As discussed in Chapters 4 and 5, BMI is not an indicator of body composition, fat mass, or health in athletes. This easily explains the lower mortality reported across positions when compared to the general population. However, when

TABLE 7.1 Standardized Mortality Rate in Former National Football League Players Compared to the General Population

Cause of Death	Observed	Expected	SMR
Overall	227	498.3	0.46**
All cancers	23	56.1	0.41**
Diseases of blood and blood-forming organs	1	3.0	0.34
Diabetes mellitus	4	10.6	0.38*
Mental, psychoneurotic, and personality disorders	2	8.8	0.23*
Diseases of the nervous system and sense organs	5	7.6	0.65
All cause cardiovascular	47	69.2	0.68**
Diseases of the circulatory system	12	21.3	0.56*
Diseases of the respiratory system	2	13.6	0.15**
Diseases of the digestive system	8	19.6	0.41**
Diseases of musculoskeletal and connective tissue	1	1.6	0.61
Diseases of the genitourinary system	1	5.8	0.17*
Transportation injuries	34	52.0	0.65*
Falls	2	3.4	0.58
Other injury (drowning, forces of nature, accidental poisoning, injuries of undetermined intent)	24	45.3	0.53**
Violence	39 (20–19)	103.3	0.38**

Source: Data adapted from Lincoln et al., 2018.

Note: SMR = standardized mortality ratio; *p < 0.05; **p < 0.01.

comparing among NFL players themselves, differences in BMI are associated with different risk patterns. Figure 7.1 shows the cardiovascular risk patterns between NFL players among themselves and versus the general population. A BMI ≥35 significantly increases the risk for cardiovascular mortality in these players compared to their leaner peers. This may actually become worse in the next few years as the number of former 300-lb players, which has increased dramatically in the past 20 years in football, reach middle-age.

In 2007, Schwenk and colleagues surveyed 3,377 former NFL players to assess the prevalence of depressive symptoms and pain as well as the difficulties with the transition from active athletic competition to retirement. The sample of subjects surveyed was obtained from the active membership list of the NFLPA, retired players section (NFLPA-RP). The mean age of all respondents was 53.4 ±14.5 years, and 80% were married. The average length of career was 7.1 ± 3.6 years, and the former players played for 2.3 ± 1.3 teams during their career. The median time since retirement was 25 years. Careers ended by being "cut" (n = 557; e.g., career ended not because of injury and not of their own choosing), "retired of my own choice" (n = 559), or retired because of a career-ending injury (n = 470). The most common problems reported by the former players in retirement can be observed in Table 7.2. The most common problem was difficulty with pain. In a questionnaire assessing depression, 14.7% of the respondents achieved a score that was defined as moderate to severe depression. Respondents scoring as moderate to severely depressed were 11.2 times more likely to report trouble sleeping than those rated as not or mildly depressed, 7.8 times more likely to report a loss of fitness and lack of exercise, and 7.1 times more likely to report financial difficulties. Other problems that were associated with respondents rated as moderately to severely depressed were lack of social support or friendships, use of prescribed medication, alcohol, or other drugs, and trouble with the transition to life after professional football. The investigators of this study indicated that the former NFL players

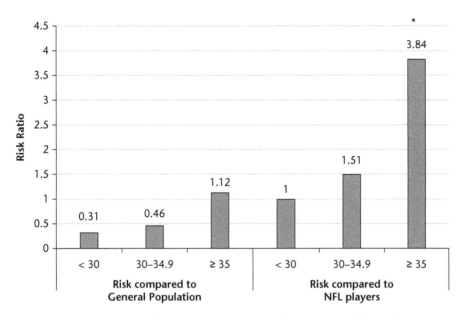

FIGURE 7.1   Cardiovascular Mortality Risk Ratio to General Population and NFL Players.

★ = significant risk compared to other groups; BMI = body mass index.

Source: Data from Lincoln et al., 2018.

TABLE 7.2 Most Common Retirement Problems in Retired NFL Players

Problem	% of Players Indicating
Pain	48
Loss of fitness and lack of exercise	29
Weight gain	28
Trouble sleeping	28
Difficulty with aging	27
Trouble with transition to life after professional football	27

Source: Data from Schwenk et al., 2007.

experienced depressive symptoms at a rate that is similar to that found in the general population; however, the former NFL players had the additional issue of substantial chronic pain. Later in this chapter the role of concussion and depression will be examined.

One of the issues often overlooked when it comes to healthy aging in former football players is that the vast majority of the literature is focused on the former professional athlete. However, they make up a very small segment of the population that played many years of competitive football. Although an argument could be made that the longer the professional career, the more likely severe medical issues will occur, there have been no difference reported in the mortality rate in players with ≥5 years playing time in the NFL compared to players who played <5 years (Lincoln et al., 2018). Considering the high injury rate observed in college football players (Kerr et al., 2016a), how these players age is also worthy of examination. There have been a limited number of studies that have examined this question. One study examined quality of life issues in former NCAA Division I athletes (Simon and Docherty, 2016). The collision sport athletes, primarily college football players, had the worst quality of life scores of any of the college athletes surveyed. They have significantly less physical function ability, greater pain, and reduced health than former athletes who participated in both collision (i.e., basketball, soccer, wresting) and limited contact (i.e., baseball, tennis, track, and field) sports.

Cardiovascular Health and Metabolic Syndrome of Retired Football Players

One of the initial studies reporting on the cardiovascular health of former NFL players examined 510 retired players were screened at several NFL player association chapter meetings over the course of 28 months (Miller et al., 2008). Comparisons were made between former linemen (n = 164, 54.0 ± 12.5 years) and skill position players (n = 346, 53.5 ± 16.5 years). Linemen played longer in the NFL (6.8 ± 3.5 years) compared to the skill position players (6.0 ± 3.7 years) and were taller, heavier, and had greater BMI and percent body fat than the skill position players. In addition, fasting glucose was higher and HDL concentrations were lower in linemen compared to the skill position players. Linemen were also more likely (p = 0.01) to be previously diagnosed for diabetes than skill players (10.4% versus 4.0%, respectively). A significantly (p < 0.001) larger percentage of linemen (67.7%) had a body fat percentage indicative of obesity compared with the former skill position players (41.9%). Metabolic syndrome was present in 59.8% of retired linemen and in only 30.1% of retired skill position players. These differences were significant (see Table 7.3). Although systolic blood pressure was significantly higher in retired linemen compared to retired skill position players, there were no differences between the groups in the percent of players whose blood pressure was ≥130 mmHg and elevated triglyceride concentrations. The investigators did not believe that obesity and its

TABLE 7.3 Comparison of Component Criteria of Metabolic Syndrome in Retired NFL Linemen and Skill Position Players

Variable	Linemen (n = 164)	Skill Position Players (n = 346)
BMI ≥ 30 kg m^{-2}	140 (85.4%)*	174 (50.3%)
Resting blood pressure ≥130 mmHg systolic and 85 mmHg diastolic	111 (67.7%)	212 (61.3%)
Reduced HDL Cholesterol ≤40 mg·dl^{-1}	69 (42.1%)*	113 (32.7%)
Elevated fasting glucose ≥100 mg·dl^{-1} or previously diagnosed type II diabetes	99 (60.4%)*	130 (37.6%)
Elevated fasting triglycerides ≥150 mg·dl^{-1}	51 (31.1%)*	83 (24.0%)
Metabolic syndrome	98 (59.8%)*	104 (30.1%)

Source: Adapted from Miller et al., 2008.

Note: Criteria for a diagnosis of metabolic syndrome was BMI ≥30 kg m^{-2} and fulfilling two or more of the other criteria. * = significant difference (p < 0.05) between groups.

metabolic consequences were of critical concern, but with increasing body size of NFL players that was becoming more common, an effort should be made for a focus on cardiovascular health and lifestyle changes in these athletes.

Concern for cardiovascular health is, in general, one that is more relevant post-career than during the athlete's career. Although the average football players are much larger than the general population and their BMI approach and exceed what would normally be considered to be obese, these men are not obese, nor are they at an elevated risk for cardiovascular disease. Tucker and colleagues (2009) reported NFL players with lower mean fasting glucose, with no significant differences in total cholesterol, LDL cholesterol, HDL cholesterol, or triglyceride concentrations, compared to age-matched controls. The only difference noted was that both systolic (127 mmHg) and diastolic (75 mmHg) blood pressures were significantly higher in the NFL players, but these levels were still considered normal. It is the lifestyle choices after their career that is of concern. Dietary habits and exercise patterns need to be changed to meet the needs of the retired athlete to focus more on health than on "bulking".

In studies comparing cardiovascular disease risk factors between former NFL players and age-matched controls, the NFL players do not appear to be at any greater risk (Chang et al., 2009; Allen et al., 2010). However, if lifestyle changes are not made by the players during their retirement years, a substantial increase in risk may be seen. Recently, a study examined the change in BMI following retirement and reported that increases in BMI are independently associated with increases in CVD, diabetes, and hypertension (Trexler et al., 2018). If the players are not careful about their weight gain, the long-term health consequence may become problematic.

Long-Term Health Consequences of Concussions in Football

In 2005, a study was published examining the effect of previous head injuries and its effect on the risk for Alzheimer's disease and mild cognitive impairment (Guskiewicz et al., 2005). Mild cognitive impairment was defined as older adults who exhibit some evidence of cognitive decline (usually in memory) and perform poorly on neurocognitive assessments, but the degree of impairment and/or functional decline do not meet the diagnostic criteria for dementia. The investigators sent a health questionnaire to all living members of the NFL's Retired Player's Association (n = 3,683). The questionnaire included questions about the number of concussions sustained during their professional football career and the prevalence of diagnosed medical conditions such as depression, Parkinson's disease, Alzheimer's disease, and schizophrenia. Previous concussion was based on the player's recall of a head injury that resulted in an alteration in mental status and one or more of the following symptoms: headache, nausea, vomiting, dizziness/balance problems, fatigue, trouble sleeping, drowsiness, sensitivity to light or noise, blurred vision, difficulty remembering, and difficulty concentrating. Four months after the initial questionnaire, the investigators sent a second questionnaire focusing on memory and issues related to cognitive function to a cohort of the original group. In addition, the second questionnaire was also sent to the spouse or close relative of the retiree to corroborate memory or cognitive impairments.

Results of the study indicated that 60.8% of the retired players completing the questionnaire sustained at least one concussion during their professional playing career, and 24% of the former players indicated that they sustained three or more concussions. More than half of the players who sustained a concussion also indicated that they experienced a loss of consciousness (54%) or memory loss (52%) from that episode. In those former players who sustained a concussion, 17.6% indicated that they believed that the concussion had a permanent effect on their thinking and memory skills as they aged. Only 1.3% of the former players had been diagnosed with Alzheimer's disease. In comparison to age-matched controls from the general population, the former football players appeared to have a greater risk for Alzheimer's disease (overall age-adjusted prevalence ratio of 1.37). In addition, the former players also had an earlier onset of the disease. However, no association was noted between the number of concussions sustained as a professional player and diagnosis of Alzheimer's disease. However, former players with a history of concussion, especially recurrent concussion, performed worse on the mental component scale scores than those who were not concussed. Players with three or more concussions scored significantly worse than age-matched controls. An association was also noted between repeated concussions and mild cognitive impairment and self-reported memory impairments and spouse/relative-reported significant memory impairments. Retired players with three or more concussions had a fivefold greater prevalence of being diagnosed with mild cognitive impairment and a threefold greater prevalence of reporting significant memory problems compared to players without a history of sustaining concussions.

As discussed earlier in this chapter, the movie "Concussion" brought to light the issues associated with the disease CTE. CTE is a neurodegenerative disease only found in individuals with a history of exposure to repetitive head impacts (McKee et al., 2010; Riley et al., 2015). CTE is characterized neuropathologically by hyperphosphorylated tau (p-tau) deposits throughout the brain, specifically in the form of neurofibrillary tangles, astrocytic tangles, and threadlike neuropil neurites (Riley et al., 2015). Exposure to repetitive brain trauma during life, including, but not limited to, the type of head impacts that may occur while playing football, or blast injury in the military has been associated with CTE neuropathology. Unfortunately, these cases are only discovered when examining brain tissue postmortem. In the initial study describing the postmortem examination of several former football players, it was found that the brain of those athletes who were not diagnosed with motor neuron disease consisted of numerous tau-positive neurofibrillary tangles, neuropil neurites, and astrocytic tangles in the frontal, temporal, and insular cortices, diencephalon, basal ganglia, and brainstem (McKee et al., 2010). In the former athletes who were previously diagnosed with motor neuron disease, the same findings were observed, except that atrophy of the ventral roots of the spinal cord were also noted (McKee et al., 2010). In interviews with the families of the deceased players, reports of either behavioral or mood changes were prominent as their initial symptoms, but there were also reports of changes in cognitive function. These symptoms generally appeared at a relatively young age (34.5 years) (Riley et al., 2015).

Dr. Ann McKee, who has been one of the most prevalent clinical scientists working on CTE, created a four-stage progression of the disease based upon her postmortem study of individuals with CTE (see Table 7.4) (McKee et al., 2013). These stages have provided a spectrum of disease progression that can provide clinicians and scientists with an understanding of the clinical and pathological features that occur after repeated brain trauma. The development of these stages was based on her team's examination of the brains of 85 donors with a history of mild traumatic brain injury, including 80 athletes (22 of whom were also military veterans), 3 military veterans with no history of contact sports, 1 civilian who had experienced multiple falls, and 1 individual who engaged in self-injurious repetitive head-banging behavior (84 males, 1 female, age range 14–98 years, mean ± SD; 54.1 ± 23.3 years). Nearly 37% of the individuals with CTE had comorbid neurodegenerative disease, including motor neuron dysfunction, Parkinson's disease, Lewy body disease, Alzheimer's disease, and frontotemporal lobar degeneration. Repetitive traumatic brain injury and axonal injury occurring during a concussive event was suggested to trigger molecular pathways that resulted in the overproduction and aggregation of proteins prone to neurodegenerative disease (McKee et al., 2013).

TABLE 7.4 Spectrum of Disease Progression in Chronic Traumatic Encephalopathy

	Major Pathological Symptoms	*Clinical Symptoms*
Stage I	• *Gross neuropathological features*: Brain weights are unremarkable • *Molecular*: p-tau pathology is restricted to discrete foci in the cerebral cortex, most commonly in the superior, dorsolateral or lateral frontal cortices, and typically around small vessels at the depths of sulci	• Can be asymptomatic • Majority report headache and loss of attention and concentration • Possible short-term memory difficulties • Aggressive tendencies and depression • Possible executive dysfunction and explosivity
Stage II	• *Gross neuropathological features*: No evidence of cerebral atrophy. Mild enlargement of the frontal horn of the lateral ventricles and a possible small cavum septum and enlargement and sharp concavity of the third ventricle • *Molecular:* There are multiple epicenters at the depths of the cerebral sulci and localized spread of neurofibrillary pathology from these epicenters to the superficial layers of adjacent cortex. The medial temporal lobe is spared neurofibrillary p-tau pathology	• Majority of individuals are symptomatic • Common presenting symptoms are depression or mood swings, headaches and short-term memory loss • May also present with symptoms of motor neuron dysfunction • May also present with symptoms of explosivity and loss of attention and concentration • Less common symptoms included executive dysfunction, impulsivity, suicidality, and language difficulties
Stage III	• *Gross neuropathological features:* Most brains showed mild cerebral atrophy with dilation of the lateral and third ventricles. Septal abnormalities were found in 42% of intact brain specimens ranging from cavum septum, septal perforations, or complete absence of the septum. Fifty-eight percent of brains showed moderate depigmentation of the locus coeruleus and 42% showed mild depigmentation of the substantia nigra. Other common gross pathological features are atrophy of the mammillary bodies and thalamus, sharply convex contour of the medial thalamus, and thinning of the hypothalamic floor and corpus callosum • *Molecular:* p-tau pathology is widespread; the frontal, insular, temporal and parietal cortices show neurofibrillary degeneration with greatest severity in the frontal and temporal lobe, concentrated at the depths of the sulci. Also, the amygdala, hippocampus, and entorhinal cortex show neurofibrillary pathology	• The most common presenting symptoms were reported to be memory loss, executive dysfunction, explosivity, and difficulty with attention and concentration • Other symptoms included depression or mood swings, visuospatial difficulties, and aggression • Less common symptoms included impulsivity, apathy, headaches, and suicidality • Cognitive impairments were noted in 75% of subjects • Possible motor neuron dysfunction after onset of behavioral and cognitive abnormalities or possible motor neuron dysfunction can occur after changes in cognitive function

(Continued)

TABLE 7.4 (Continued)

	Major Pathological Symptoms	Clinical Symptoms
Stage IV	• *Gross neuropathological features:* Brain changes included atrophy of the cerebral cortex and white matter and marked atrophy of the medial temporal lobe, thalamus, hypothalamus, and mammillary body. Mean brain weight was significantly smaller than lower stage CTE. Most brains showed ventricular enlargement, a sharply concave contour of the third ventricle, septal perforations, or septal absence. Pallor of the locus coeruleus and substantia nigra were found in all instances where it could be assessed • *Molecular:* There is severe p-tau pathology affecting most regions of the cerebral cortex and the medial temporal lobe, sparing calcarine cortex in all but the most severe cases	• All subjects were symptomatic • Executive dysfunction and memory loss were the most common symptoms at onset, and all developed severe memory loss with dementia during their course • Most subjects also showed profound loss of attention and concentration, executive dysfunction, language difficulties, explosivity, aggressive tendencies, paranoia, depression, gait, and visuospatial difficulties • Less common symptoms were impulsivity, dysarthria, and Parkinsonism; 31% were suicidal at some point in their course • A small percentage of individuals developed symptoms of motor neuron dysfunction years after developing cognitive and behavioral abnormalities

Source: Adapted from McKee et al., 2013.

A subsequent autopsy study examined 202 brains of deceased former American football players who ranged in playing experience from high school, college, semiprofessional, and professional levels (Mez et al., 2017). A high proportion of the brains of these former athletes had a neuropathological assessment consistent with CTE. The severity of CTE pathology was distributed across the highest level of play, with all former high school players having mild pathology and the majority of former college, semiprofessional, and professional players having severe pathology. In discussions with family members, the investigators were able to understand the former players' behavior, mood, and cognitive function. The behavioral and cognitive dysfunction was noted in those with mild and severe CTE pathology and signs of dementia were common among those with severe CTE pathology. Nearly all of the former NFL players examined in this study had CTE pathology, and this pathology was frequently severe. The most unique finding of this study was the suggestion that CTE may be related to prior participation in football. Thus, even high school football participation may be sufficient to cause symptoms and pathology related to CTE. A greater disease progression though was seen in the former NFL players, although this is more likely related to greater concussive events that would occur over a longer career.

There have been a number of publications that have examined the effect of age of *first exposure* and subsequent risk for brain injury and neurodysfunction (Alosco et al., 2017a, 2018; Stamm et al., 2015). Stamm and colleagues (2015) examined 66 former NFL players. Inclusion criterion for this study was that they had to play organized football for at least 12 years and played at least 2 years in the NFL. In addition, participants must have had a worsening of cognitive, behavioral, and mood symptoms for at least the last 6 months or they have received treatment from a doctor for these symptoms. These symptoms included difficulties with memory, planning and organization, impulsivity, violence, depression, anxiety, and/or apathy. Participants were categorized into two groups: those who were first exposed to organized football before the age of 12 (n = 30, 50.3 ± 6.6 years), and those who were exposed to organized football after the age of 12 (n = 36, 57.4 ± 7.4 years). All former players participated in a magnetic resonance imaging (MRI) procedure called diffusion tensor imaging (DTI). DTI is an advanced MRI technique that provides information regarding the brain's white matter microstructure by measuring the magnitude and direction of water molecules (Basser and Pierpaoli, 1996). The directionality of this diffusion is commonly measured using fractional anisotropy (FA). A higher FA value is indicative of a greater diffusion along one direction, as would be expected in well-organized, intact tissue (Song et al., 2002). In poorly organized tissues, the multidirectional movement of water molecules can occur with little resistance. Other common diffusion measures include axial (AD) and radial (RD) diffusivity, which are thought to measure axonal and myelin pathology, respectively (Song et al., 2002). Stamm and colleagues (2015) reported that former NFL players who started playing tackle football prior to age 12 had lower FA values and greater RD in anterior corpus callosum regions, compared with those who started playing football at age 12 or older. Exposure to repeated head trauma during a critical period of neurodevelopment may disrupt normal axonal maturation and myelination, leading to permanently altered white matter microstructure. Others have reported that former players who began to play before the age of 12 had more than a twofold greater risk for behavioral impairment, apathy, and reduced executive function and more than a threefold greater risk for experiencing clinically elevated depression scores when compared to former players who began playing after the age of 12 (Alosco et al., 2017a).

In a postmortem examination of both amateur and professional football players whose brains were donated, Alosco and colleagues (2018) examined the effect of age at first organized football exposure and stage of CTE. Their investigation revealed no association between age of first exposure to organized football and CTE pathological severity. However, a younger start to organized tackle football was able to predict behavioral and mood changes. For every year younger than 12 that a former player began to play football was related to an earlier onset of cognitive and behavioral/mood symptoms by approximately 2.5 years. Beginning to play tackle football before the age of 12 corresponded to an earlier onset of cognitive impairment by 12.4 years and behavioral and mood symptoms by 13.3 years. These findings were independent of level or duration of play.

Neuroimaging and Biomarkers for Identification of Neurological Issues in Former Players

The only way to determine whether a former player has CTE is through a postmortem autopsy. At present, there is no biomarker or other noninvasive imaging procedure that has proven validity. However, there has been much effort exploring various invasive and noninvasive possibilities. The examination of circulating concentrations of plasma total (t)-tau concentrations has been examined as a potential biomarker (Alosco et al., 2017b). The investigators recruited 124 subjects (96 former NFL players and 28 age-matched controls). Study participants were required to be former NFL players, aged 40–69 years, with a minimum of two seasons in the NFL and a minimum of 12 years playing organized football, and had self-reported complaints of cognitive, behavioral, and/or mood symptoms at the time of recruitment. The former players were also required to not have had a history of concussion within one year before the study enrollment. The age-matched control group was required to have no history of participation in contact sports, no military service, and no self-reported traumatic brain injury (TBI) or concussion history, including no cognitive, behavioral, and/or mood symptoms at the time of recruitment. Nonfasting blood samples were collected in both groups. Results of the study indicated that greater exposure to repetitive head impacts during the former NFL athlete's playing career was associated with elevated plasma t-tau concentrations later in life (Alosco et al., 2017b). However, no differences in plasma t-tau concentrations were noted between the former NFL players and age-matched controls. There were a number of former NFL players who exhibited more extreme plasma t-tau concentrations, with 12.5% of the players having plasma t-tau concentrations >3.56 $pg \cdot ml^{-1}$ (the highest t-tau concentration was 6.19 $pg \cdot ml^{-1}$). No participant in the control group had plasma t-tau concentrations >3.56 $pg \cdot ml^{-1}$, making this concentration 100% specific to the former NFL players, and any former player with a plasma t-tau concentration >3.56 $pg \cdot ml^{-1}$ also had significantly greater exposure to repeated head trauma compared to former players with plasma t-tau concentrations below 3.56 $pg \cdot ml^{-1}$.

Other biomarkers that have been examined include calpain-derived αII-spectrin N-terminal fragment (SNTF), which is another marker for axonal injury. Serum SNTF concentrations have been reported to be elevated from 1 h up to six days post-concussion in professional ice-hockey players post-injury (Siman et al., 2015). S100B is an astrocyte-enriched Ca^{2+} binding protein. Although it has been proposed to be a potential marker for mild traumatic brain injury (Oris et al., 2018), it has yet to be examined in active or former football players. Others have suggested that S100B may not be sensitive enough to detect brain injury in concussion (Schulte et al., 2014). Glial fibrillary acidic protein (GFAP) is an intermediate filament that is almost exclusively expressed in astrocytes. GFAP concentration is highly specific in brain tissue and is regarded as a sensitive and reliable marker of neuroinflammation and brain injury (Hiskens et al., 2020. It has also been suggested to be a marker for acute mild traumatic brain injury from sport (McCrea et al., 2020), but it has not yet been examined in regard to retired football players and brain health.

There have also been several studies using neuroimaging in an attempt to determine risk for CTE. Investigators have used positron emission tomography, magnetic resonance spectroscopy (MRS), MRI, functional MRI, and DTI. Although there is benefit for each one of these devices, a recent review paper on neuroimaging techniques and CTE suggests that the most successful method to detect and diagnose CTE and other long-term consequences of repeated head injury in football or other contact/collision sports will utilize a multimodal neuroimaging approach (Lin et al., 2018). One study recruited former college and professional football players without any known cognitive impairment to perform several imaging protocols involving both DTI and functional MRI measures (Clark et al., 2018). Investigators recorded the players' previous concussion history. Results indicated an interesting effect of concussion history on white matter integrity and functional neural recruitment. In the college-only cohort, those athletes with more than three concussions during their career had a lower FA than those with zero to one concussion in their career. However, in a surprising result, the former NFL players who reported multiple concussions had a higher FA than the former NFL players with zero to one concussion. This could have been a spurious outcome or may represent a measure of resiliency in this group of former athletes, who were not cognitively affected. This was consistent with other studies that reported no differences in FA in former NFL players without any behavioral abnormalities compared to age-matched controls (Hart et al., 2013; Goswami et al., 2016; Strain et al., 2013). In addition, there were no significant interactions observed between concussion history and career duration in the functional MR imaging blood oxygen level-dependent (BOLD) data for any condition contrast.

In a study of former NFL players, Lepage and colleagues (2019) compared the volumes of the amygdala, hippocampus, and cingulate gyrus in symptomatic former NFL players relative to asymptomatic controls without a history of repeated head injury or brain trauma. The investigators also examined the association between regions of volume reduction and neurocognitive and behavioral functioning in the former players. Former NFL players were between 40 and 69 years of age, with at least 12 years of organized football experience and 2 or more years of active participation in the NFL and self-reported declines in cognition, mood, and behavior within 6 months of study enrollment. Participants in the control group were of similar age with no behavioral or cognitive issues. The former symptomatic NFL players exhibited reduced volumes of the amygdala, hippocampus, and cingulate gyrus regions compared to controls. In addition, the lower volumes within the limbic system structures were associated with reduced neurocognitive function.

Alosco and colleagues (2019) used MRS to examine neurochemical concentrations in symptomatic former NFL players. They were interested in examining the relationship between repeated head injury and neurochemistry and between the associations among neurochemistry and neuropsychological and neuropsychiatric functioning. Results of the study indicated that in the former NFL players, a higher cumulative head impact index (an index of repeated head impacts that was estimated) was significantly correlated with creatine concentrations in the parietal lobe white matter ($r = -0.23$, $p = 0.02$). No other significant relationship was observed between head impact index and other neuronal viability measures (i.e., N-acetyl aspartate, glutamate/glutamine, choline, myo-inositol, and glutathione). In comparison to age-matched asymptomatic controls without a history of head trauma, the former NFL players exhibited significantly lower parietal white matter N-acetyl aspartate levels, but no other differences were noted. The anterior cingulate gyrus was the only brain area that was shown to be associated with clinical function. Significant positive correlations ($p < 0.05$) were observed between N-acetyl aspartate ($r = 0.42$), glutamate ($r = 0.32$), glutathione ($r = 0.29$), and myo-inositol ($r = 0.26$) concentrations in the anterior cingulate gyrus and behavioral/mood composite scores. A higher score on the behavioral mood composition was considered a poorer behavioral outcome. In addition, significant correlations were also noted between glutamate/glutamine ratio ($r = 0.24$) in the anterior cingulate gyrus and psychomotor speed/executive function, and between creatine ($r = 0.27$) and glutamate ($r = 0.26$) concentrations in the anterior cingulate gyrus with visual memory. This investigation found a direct relationship between repeated head exposure and reductions in cellular metabolism as measured by MRS technology. In addition, changes in neuroinflammatory markers in the anterior cingulate gyrus may have important clinical information regarding behavior and mood disturbances in players with a history of concussion.

Relationship Between Concussion History and Depression in Former Players

Earlier in this chapter, the relationship between previous head injuries and cognitive function in former NFL players was described (Guskiewicz et al., 2005). That large study produced several other interesting data sets as well. In 2007, the investigative teams published another paper examining the effect of previous head injuries and depression (Guskiewicz et al., 2007). In their analysis of the questionnaires completed by the former players, they identified 11% of the 2,434 respondents with complete data sets as having been diagnosed with clinical depression. Those former players with diagnosed depression had lower mental component scores on the SF-36 compared to former players who were not clinically depressed. In addition, a linear association was observed between concussion history and the diagnosis of depression. Former players reporting a history of one or two previous concussions were 1.5 times more likely to have been diagnosed with depression, and former players with a history of three or more previous concussions were 3 times more likely to be diagnosed with depression than former players

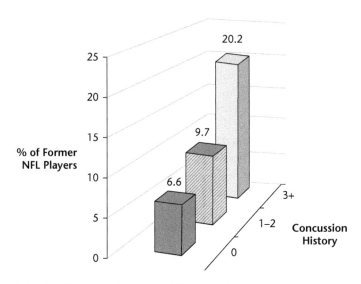

FIGURE 7.2 Relationship Between Concussion History and Depression.

Source: Data from Guskiewicz et al., 2007.

with no history of concussion (see Figure 7.2). The relationship between concussion history and depression was still similar even when the investigators controlled for mild cognitive impairments among the players.

In a follow-up study, Kerr and colleagues (2012) examined nine years of data (2001–2010) in the former NFL players. Some of these players began their career prior to World War II, while others played in the new millennium. There were 1,044 respondents, of which 106 (10.2%) were diagnosed as being clinically depressed. Of these 106 respondents, 68 (64.2%) reported still suffering from depression in 2010, and 36 (34.0%) were currently being treated with antidepressant medications. A total of 365 (35.0%) former players indicated that they were not concussed during their professional career, 25.8% reported one to two concussions, 19.5% reported three to four concussions, 12.9% self-reported five to nine concussions, and 6.8% indicated that they were concussed ten or more times. The nine-year risk of a depression diagnosis increased with increasing number of self-reported concussions, ranging from 3.0% in the "no concussion" group to 26.8% in the 10+ group. The percentage of players reporting concussion and relative risk for depression can be observed in Figure 7.3. Similar to the previous study by Guskiewicz et al. (2007), the greater number of concussions recalled in one's career resulted in a greater risk for depression. The linear dose–response relationship was confirmed.

Are There Other Medical Risks Associated With Concussion?

Tarazi and colleagues (2018) examined the effect of concussion history on motor function in former professional football players. Forty-five former Canadian Football League (CFL) players (53.4 ± 10.3 years) with an average concussion history of 5.1 ± 4.2 concussion per player were compared to age-matched controls without any concussion history. The time since last concussion in the former players was 17.3 ± 14.8 years. No differences were observed in self-reported motor symptoms between the two groups. In addition, no differences were noted in motor coordination assessment using the grooved pegboard test between the former CFL players and

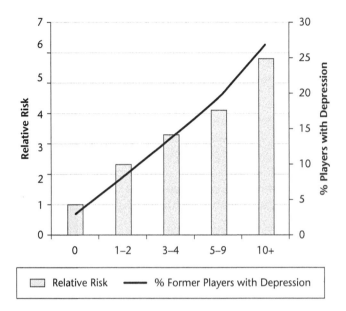

FIGURE 7.3 Effect of Concussion History on Relative Risk for Depression.

Source: Data from Kerr et al., 2012.

control subjects in their dominant (45.29 versus 46.92, p = 0.57, respectively) or nondominant (77.7 versus 81.2, p = 0.48) hands. However, significant differences were noted between the groups on memory, executive function, and behavioral symptoms in the group of former CFL players compared to the control group. Similar to previous reports, concussion was associated with changes to behavior, although the results of this study indicated that concussion history does not appear to influence motor impairment.

Others have examined whether injury history, including concussion, was associated with osteoarthritis in former NFL players (Lynall et al., 2017). The survey was sent to former NFL players and 2,696 of the former players responded. Of the respondents, 36.3% reported experiencing osteoarthritis (OA) during their lifetime. Of the former players experiencing OA, 40.1% reported no concussion history, 19.4% experienced one concussion, 16.3% reported experiencing two concussions, and 24.2% reported a history of three or more concussions. A diagnosis of OA was associated with the number of lower extremity body injuries, ranging from 26.1% for no lower extremity injuries to 29.6% for one lower extremity injury and 44.4% for two or more lower extremity injuries. The prevalence of OA in former athletes with two or more lower extremity injuries was 70% greater than that in athletes with no previous injuries. Former athletes older than 55 years had a greater prevalence for OA than younger former players. Interestingly, the number of concussions sustained during one's career may also be related to OA. Former players with multiple concussions demonstrated a greater prevalence of OA than those with zero or one concussion. Former NFL athletes who had two or more lower extremity injuries with three or more concussion had the greater risk for OA (50.6% of the athletes reported having OA).

Concussion history has also been reported to be related to reduced testosterone concentrations (Grashow et al., 2019) and pituitary function (Kelly et al., 2014) in former NFL players. Chronic hypopituitarism has been reported in 23.5% of former football players (Kelly et al.,

2014). Although it was noted that players averaged approximately three concussions each, the relationship between concussion history and pituitary function was not analyzed. Grashow and colleagues (2019) specifically examined testosterone concentrations and erectile dysfunction (ED) in former NFL players. Low testosterone concentration was observed in 18.3% of 3,506 former NFL players, and 22.7% of the former players reported symptoms that were indicators of ED. The investigators also reported that only 9.8% of the former players reported both low testosterone concentrations and ED. In models that included age and race, Grashow and colleagues (2019) also indicated that low testosterone concentrations and ED were significantly associated with hypertension, high cholesterol concentrations, diabetes, CVD, prescription pain medication, reproductive cancer, sleep apnea, obesity, and mood disorders. Examining the effect of concussion on testosterone concentrations and ED, Grasham and colleagues (2019) reported that the greater frequency of concussion (highest quartile of occurrence) during one's playing career was associated with low testosterone concentrations and ED during the former players' retirement.

What Is the Risk for Neurodegenerative Disease in Former Football Players?

Much of this chapter has been focused on the health of former NFL players. Although some investigations included former college players, little information is available on former high school only players. Is high school football playing experience associated with any increased risk for impaired aging? This is especially relevant as CTE has also been linked to individuals who played high school football only (McKee et al., 2013). The effect of high school football on neurodegenerative function was examined in a cohort of former players who had participated when protective headgear was not optimal and that players were expected to play through concussive hits (Savica et al., 2012). These investigators examined athletes who played during 1946–1956. Because CTE has been linked to neurodegenerative diseases such as dementia, Alzheimer's disease, and Parkinson's disease, they specifically examined these three conditions. They compared their sample to an age-matched control group that did not participate in any sports activity, but had gone to the same high school, and to age-adjusted incident rates of these diseases within the general population. A total of 438 former football players and 140 high school colleagues were analyzed via medical records. No significant differences were noted between the former players and nonathletes in regard to risk for dementia, Parkinson's disease, or amyotrophic lateral sclerosis (see Table 7.5). The results did not support a greater risk for neurodegenerative disease for individuals who played high school football only. A follow-up study examining athletes of a later decade (1956–1970) also found no greater risk for neurodegenerative diseases in later life from high school football playing experience (Janssen et al., 2017).

Playing duration does appear to have an effect on neurodegenerative disease. In a study on former NFL players, the duration of time played and position played were associated with lasting neuropsychiatric health deficits later in life (Roberts et al., 2019). Career length and playing position in the NFL have been shown to be associated with poor cognition-related quality of life (QOL), depression, and anxiety in a large sample of former players. Analysis of 3,506 former players who had played in the NFL since 1960 was conducted. Respondents had a mean age of 52.8 ± 14.2 years and the median number of years for the group since last playing was 24 years. Cognition-related QOL was associated with seasons of professional play and playing position. Of the former players who played only one season, 5.8% had poor cognition-related QOL versus 12.6% of men who played more than one season. Positional comparisons for QOL, depression, and anxiety can be examined in Table 7.6. Running backs, defensive linemen, and linebackers were at elevated risk of poor cognition-related QOL as compared with kickers/punters. The

TABLE 7.5 Risk of Neurodegenerative Disease in Former High School Football Players

	Former High School Football Players (n = 438)	Age-Matched Controls (n = 140)	Hazard Risk
Dementia	3.0%	1.4%	1.58
Parkinson's disease	2.3%	3.6%	0.48
Amyotrophic lateral sclerosis	0.5%	0.7%	0.52

Source: Adapted from Savica et al., 2012.

TABLE 7.6 Effect of Playing Position on Risk of Poor Cognition-Related Quality of Life, Indicators of Depression, and Indicators of Anxiety in Players With Former NFL Players

	Poor Cognition-Related Quality of Life	Indicators of Depression	Indicators of Anxiety
Kicker/punters	1.0	1.0	1.0
Quarterbacks	1.42	1.21	0.97
Wide receivers	2.06	1.19	1.28
Tight ends	1.60	1.28	0.93
Running backs	3.64*	2.07*	1.82*
Offensive linemen	2.31	1.68	1.47
Linebackers	2.84*	1.50	1.28
Defensive backs	1.87	1.36	1.26
Defensive linemen	2.71*	1.91*	1.57*

Source: Data from Roberts et al., 2019.

Notes: * = significant from kickers/punters $p < 0.05$. The kickers/punters served as the reference value. Risk was adjusted for age and race.

kickers/punters served as the reference value. Responses of the former NFL players indicated that 23.9% and 25.9% of the former players were suffering from depression and anxiety, respectively, and 18.3% of the players had both. Each five years of playing experience was associated with a 9% increased risk of having depression. Depression and anxiety were associated with playing position, with running backs and defensive linemen at higher risk compared to kickers/punters. Duration of career was not associated with any change in anxiety. The investigators also examined the effect of concussion history. Player concussion symptom history was divided into quartiles. Those players in the highest quartile had a 22.3-fold greater risk of poor cognition-related QOL, 6.0-fold greater risk of depression, and 6.4-fold greater risk of anxiety compared to the lowest quartile. When risk for QOL, depression, and anxiety was adjusted for concussion symptoms, the association of seasons of play and playing position was attenuated. Thus, running backs, defensive linemen, and linebackers without any history of concussion symptoms were not at any greater risk for cognition-related QOL, depression, or anxiety.

What Is the Risk of Osteoarthritis (OA) in Former Football Players?

Arthritis comprises more than 100 medical conditions that affect joints, and OA is the most common form of arthritis. In 2009, the faculty at the University of North Carolina examined the prevalence of arthritis in former NFL players and compared their outcomes with the prevalence of OA in the general US male population (Golightly et al., 2009). The average age of the former players was 53.8 years (range: 24–95 years), and they played an average of 6.6 years (range 1–26 years) of professional football. Compared with players without OA, players with OA were older, had higher BMIs, and had poorer health status on the physical and mental health components of the SF-36. Linemen had a higher prevalence of OA compared with linebackers and running backs. Other positions were less likely to report prevalence of OA. Players with OA were more likely to report CVD, diabetes, and depression than those without OA. Overall, 43.4% of the former players reported a physician diagnosis of any type of arthritis, and 37.9% reported a physician diagnosis of OA. Arthritis was more common in the former players under the age of 60 years compared to a similar age group of the general population (40.6% versus 11.7%, respectively). As the players aged, the disparity between older former players (>60 years) and age-matched general population became much closer (49.2% versus 41.9%, respectively). The arthritis prevalence ratio in the former players was 2.5 in those under 60 years of age. The prevalence ratio was even higher in the younger age groups: 4.5 in those under 50 years and 6.5 in those under 40 years. The results of this study indicate that former NFL players are at a greater risk for OA in their middle-age years than age-matched controls. A recent study among former NFL players indicated that a history of ankle injuries had long-term negative effects on joint health and was associated with impairment of daily activities. In addition, a higher prevalence of OA was noted in retired NFL players with ankle injuries who underwent surgical intervention at the ankle or foot (Song et al., 2019).

Summary

Despite empirical belief that former football players are more prone to neurodegeneration, depression, arthritis, and cardiovascular disease, the evidence simply does not support that when comparing older former professional football players to age-matched controls. However, evidence does suggest an earlier onset of medical issues in middle-age former players who are reflective of the sport, especially those related to OA and concussion-related behavioral/cognitive issues. If a former player can make it to retirement age, health issues generally do not differ from the general population. Further, there is some evidence that some former professional players may have a resiliency toward behavioral changes related to concussion. This was an interesting finding that deserves further study. To date, CTE can only be diagnosed upon death. However, not all brains that have been examined and found to have CTE have been associated with concussive effects. Most of the research on CTE has focused on former professional football players and soldiers who had experienced repeated occurrences of mild traumatic brain injury from either concussive effects from a game or blast injury in combat. The associated symptoms during their lives and the findings on autopsy make it easy to create the link between brain injury and CTE. However, it does not establish a cause and effect.

This is a bit controversial, but perhaps needs to be debated. Football is a gladiator sport. The men who play the game love the contact. You can't be successful and play a long time if it didn't excite them. Some players are now retiring early to avoid the risk of brain injury, but this is likely a function of the economics of today's game, where the earning power of players are much different than in previous generations. Some players may realize that they have a good financial head start and move on to their next endeavor. No different than a gambler who is satisfied with his winnings for the evening and walks away and cashes in his chips. To play the game and enjoy it requires a special type of person. The average person is not willing to drive their car into a wall 60–70 times a day. That is what playing a football game feels like. So the question is whether this type of behavior is predicated on a specific chemical makeup in the brain, or is it a behavioral pattern that results from social adaptation. Recent study has suggested that behavioral genetics and epigenetics may have an important role in modulating vulnerability to proactive and reactive aggressive behavior (Palumbo et al., 2018). Whether a football player is genetically more prone for this sport is an interesting question, and if so, that may explain the autopsy findings of brains of football players with signs of CTE, but without the concussive or behavioral history. Further research is warranted in this area.

8

COACHING ASPECTS ASSOCIATED WITH AMERICAN FOOTBALL

Introduction

In contrast to the other chapters in this book, this chapter is based primarily on my experiences as a player, coach, and sport scientist since 1976. Coaching is not a quantitative science in the way physiology or chemistry is. Although statistics and probabilities often play a major role in the decision-making processes and game planning, most coaching decisions are qualitative in nature. A coach's perception, his social environment, his personal experiences all factor in his decision-making processes. There are times when the football coach needs to rely on science such as the strength and conditioning program and player recruitment and selection. Player injury and risk for injury is based more on medical evaluation and would be best appreciated with a background in science. When examining a football program in its entirety, the inclusion of both qualitative and quantitative parameters is critical for the success of the program. To justify why a coach decided to go for it on 4th and 4 on his own 45 yard line is open for debate, but for the most part that decision is based on the coach's intuition, his instinct, his desire to take a risk, and his belief in his team. However, there are actual statistical analyses and published data that a coach can rely upon and use a more scientific approach in decision-making on the field (Ferguson, 2018; Owens and Roach, 2018; Wright, 2007).

The head football coach has ultimate responsibility for the decisions made by his assistant coaches, including the strength and conditioning staff. No different than a chief executive officer (CEO) or executive director of any major organization, the head football coach is the team's CEO and has to take responsibility and be accountable for the actions of his assistants and his players. This is for any level of play and where knowledge of sport science becomes very important. Off-season conditioning programs are often used, correctly and unfortunately incorrectly, to set the tone for the upcoming season. It is for this reason that the coach needs to understand the limitations of conditioning programs. Well-designed training programs that are based upon sound science can enhance strength, size, and power of the athlete. However, it will not make a slow athlete fast, nor a timid athlete tough. That is a recruiting issue, not a strength and conditioning issue. Too many coaches have allowed, condoned, or insisted on inappropriate conditioning programs to be conducted on their teams with the purpose of "setting a tone" that resulted in the death of an athlete (Parsons et al., 2019). The idea of using exercise in a punitive manner is wrong and dangerous.

My perspective on coaching is through the prism of a player, a coach, and a sport scientist. I have played for and worked for coaches who were geniuses and have been recognized for their greatness by their profession. I worked with Jim Calhoun and Geno Auriemma, both Hall-of-Famers in College basketball. I also played for Steve Spurrier, who is in the College Football Hall-of-Fame as both a player and a coach, and I also had an interesting experience being David Blatt's first assistant coach in his first professional coaching job with Hapoel Galil Elyion in Israel. David is only the second coach in history (after Dusan Ivkovic) who has won a Euroleague championship, EuroBasket Championship, EuroCup, and Olympic medal (bronze with Russia in 2012), and he coached the Cleveland Cavaliers to the NBA Finals. On the flip side of those great coaches, I have also played or worked with coaches who were to say the least were more characters, than men of character, and I have experienced everything in-between. I can say that I have learned from everyone, things to do and also what not to do.

When you are in a leadership position, your response, behavior, and actions will always be judged. Coaches should be concerned with how they are perceived by others, but realize that they should first be okay with the man in mirror. The most important thing is to be true to your principles. A quote from Saint John Chrysostom, "Every man is the painter and the sculptor of his own life", was provided to every player at the St. John's University's football program. It is a pretty powerful message in that we control our actions and are responsible for our destiny. Talent is subjective, it is in the eyes of the beholder, similar to beauty, but work ethic, passion, and determination, these are impressions that should always be strived to be recognized. Coaches and players need to always consider that someone is always watching you for the first time. What will they say of your effort, your passion? You can lose to a better opponent, but it doesn't stop you from competing and providing your very best effort at all times. If you are able get your players to understand that, you have a good chance of achieving the success you desire.

When a coach is hired, or for that matter any person, what is the impression that you want your players, staff, and management to receive. There is only one opportunity to make a first impression. If it wasn't positive, it would take much longer to change that impression. Your organization, communication, and, most importantly, the ability to adapt will be tested. All that was promised may not always be delivered. How do you respond? From day 1, being organized, stating your expectations from those who work for you, and making adjustments to what the management was able to provide enhance your ability to successfully compete.

Coaching Education and Certification

Football coaches generally are required to have a college degree, and many have a master's degree. Although a master's degree is not required per se, often times the first opportunity to coach college football is as a graduate assistant. There is no information known regarding degree completion and degree majors among football coaches. Although there are few specific sport coaching majors available in North American Universities, many students wishing to become a football coach choose to major in a Kinesiology program that may be called Exercise Science, Sport Science, or perhaps Physical Education. The only coaching position that has a specific major is the Strength and Conditioning Coach. The National Strength and Conditioning Association (NSCA) is the largest certifying body for strength and conditioning coaches. To be certified by the NSCA, one needs a sports science degree or its equivalent. Most strength and conditioning positions require their applicants to be certified and to maintain their certification with continuing education. However, there is no such program for the football coach. Thus, it is not surprising that the range of academic experience is quite varied among football coaches.

Considering that coaching success is dependent upon the physiological performance of his athletes, it is shocking that there are no minimal standards requested from NCAA, NFL, or even high school federations. It would make sense that any coach would benefit from knowledge in exercise physiology, motor development, nutrition, sport psychology, or biomechanics. The most valuable commodity that they control is their athlete, and their knowledge of how this athlete functions is very limited. The NCAA only requires coaches to become certified on the rules of recruiting. The lack of educational requirements has been an issue raised by major sports medicine and sport science governing bodies, whose interest is in the health and welfare of the student-athlete (Casa et al., 2012). Considering the inherent injury risk associated with playing football (see Chapters 6 and 7), it is more than surprising that football coaches are not required to demonstrate a minimal knowledge base in order to be hired. This may go a long way in protecting the health of the players.

A basic lack of fundamental knowledge can turn an unfortunate event into a catastrophic one. A few years ago, a high school football player suffered a heat injury during unofficial summer practices. No athletic trainer was present and the head football coach and his assistants were on the field. They were local firemen with a high school degree only. When the player collapsed, several parents wanted to place the collapsed athlete in a cold water bath. The coach indicated that would be a mistake and prevented the parents from carrying this out. It was this simple decision, because of a lack of knowledge, that turned an unfortunate event into a catastrophic event and resulted in the player's death from heatstroke. If the player would have survived by being placed in the bath, we'll never know, but that is the initial treatment response when heatstroke is a possibility (McDermott et al., 2009). With the coach having no higher education background, was he prepared for such an event? Most likely not – even though he was a first responder, his job as a fireman did not require a knowledge base on how to treat this specific incident.

Coaching certification is a concept accepted in almost every country in the world, except the United States. What makes this issue even more concerning is the level of knowledge among coaches generally increases with the level of play, and the most vulnerable football populations (e.g., Pop Warner leagues and high school football) likely have the least prepared coaches. In Pop Warner football, it is generally the parents who are volunteering, and in high school football, it may be the math teacher who is one of the football coaches, if not the head coach. It is a complicated issue, because of the lack of funding to pay coaches in Pop Warner and the staff required of high school programs may not have a sufficient number of physical education teachers, other qualified teachers, or community members with the necessary knowledge skills are thus utilized. A possible solution is to prevent tackle football in Pop Warner football until players are past their 13th birthday. If you recall from Chapter 7, there is pretty strong evidence regarding the danger of an early start to playing organized football (Alosco et al., 2017a, 2018; Stamm et al., 2015).

Coach, Teacher, Mentor, Father

Between 2000 and 2007, I coached at the College of New Jersey (TCNJ), the last five years I was the defensive coordinator. From 2003, I also served as Department Chair of the Health and Exercise Science Program. This was a unique opportunity that few professors experience. Many of the students I taught also played on the football team. It was a great honor to wear those two hats, but what really struck me was how these student-athletes responded to me in the classroom and in the halls. All my students would refer to me as Dr. Hoffman, but the football players would always refer to me as Coach Hoffman. Even to this day, nearly 20 years later former players, even those who were my students will still call me coach. At the beginning, I didn't know how to react to this. I earned the right to be called Dr. and I was named a coach, there was no dissertation, no thesis, no exam – it was simply a position that I was hired for. I didn't understand or in the beginning appreciate the title. In time, I learned that it was a title of respect, and to this day those players who are now in their late 30s and early 40s, with their own families, still call me coach when we meet. I learned that the title of coach comes with opportunity and responsibility. The opportunity is the chance to become a mentor of a young man and help him grow into being an adult. Teaching is not just the technique involved in playing the game, but it is the confidence you build by the challenges that you set, the discipline that you provide by demanding hard work and sacrifice, the love and appreciation that you demonstrate by acknowledging effort for a job well done. It was important for me that the players would know that I was there for them and I cared about their success. Those lessons would be taught in some of the simplest drills. Learning to do the small things correctly and attention to details are all key parts in the development of the athlete and team.

When you become a coach, you have taken on a responsibility that is greater than yourself. You have agreed to become a teacher, a mentor, and at times you may be a father. You may be coaching players who lack a father figure at home. You, whether you want to or not, may be that player's only chance to have a strong male influence in his life. You can influence not just his football career, but his path in life, you can be the example that he needs to develop his own dreams. This is a huge responsibility and, most importantly, a tremendous reward if you allow it to be. Relish it, your ability to influence this player, it may put him on the right track in life. There is a Talmudic saying that *if you save a life, it is as if you saved the world*. For that player, providing that influence can have that level of impact.

There is a tremendous opportunity for coaches at the high school and collegiate levels to influence the maturation of their players. This is to be especially relevant at the high school and Division III level of football. Players participating in Division III football play because of their love of the game, there are no scholarships and their coaches' coach for the love of the game. That perspective is much different than what might be found at the Division I level. There is no doubt that coaches and players both love the game at the Division I level as well, but it is the financial disparity that may create an issue. Coaches receive it and the players do not. The salary range for head football coaches in the NCAA Division I top 25 football programs in 2019 ranged from $4.4 million to more than $9.3 million per year (Crabtree-Hannigan, 2020). In contrast, the salary for Division III coaches are not published, but the Bureau of Labor Statistics estimates the average salary of football college coaches to be little more than $43,000 per year, depending on location. The ability of Division I coaches to continue to be paid a very nice salary is dependent upon their players; that is where the potential problems begin and end. At the Division III level, the players know that they are students first and football players second. They come to the University to get an education, prepare for a professional career outside of sport, but get to extend their playing career for another four years. Although players do get to the next level from Division III football, it is quite rare. Division III football provides an interesting perspective. When the player is off the field, the expectation is to focus on his academics and be the best student he can be. Coaches receive zero bonuses or compensation on player retention or graduation rate, which is an expected part of their job responsibilities. However, as soon as the player crosses the white lines onto the football field, it is only about football. Missed practices or coming late to practice because of chemistry lab or biology lab is by no means ideal, but it is part of the norm and accepted. However, once on the field, there is no doubt regarding player effort.

At the Division I level, a player missing practice for a lab would not be acceptable. There are academic advisors who are paid specifically to ensure that these players are available for all football-related meetings/practices or training sessions. Players may not have the freedom to major in anything they want, if it interferes with practice times. An argument is often made in that many of these players are in college to prepare for their chosen profession: professional football – no different than a pre-med or a pre-law major. That appears to be a straw man argument.

In contrast to the pre-med and pre-law majors, which are also ultracompetitive, these students do have a specific major to rely on if medical or law school admission is not successful. I have also been shocked at the attitude of some coaches at the Division I level in regard to their expectations from their scholarship athletes. I was in a meeting regarding safety in college football, after a rash of off-season deaths. One of the strength coaches at the meeting insisted that "the players owe the program to work hard". The meeting included physicians, athletic trainers, football coaches, strength and conditioning coaches, academics, and an attorney. When this particular coach finished his diatribe, I told one of the physicians and the attorney that he will eventually kill someone. Within a year, a player died in his program from overuse during the off-season conditioning practice. No one doubts the necessity of hard work, but pushing yourself to your limit is much different than being pushed by a coach past your limit. Coaches need to realize the importance of what they say and how it impacts their players. Coach Jim Calhoun, the Hall-of-Fame basketball coach, explained once the difference between the reaction from his players to him saying something versus his assistants; "it's very simple, I hold 200 minutes in my hand, and I can divide them up any which way I'd like". All of those players want to get to the next level, and the only way they can get there is earning those minutes. That is a tremendous responsibility for the coach. When you have that type of influence, what do you do? What message do you want to send? What behavior do you reward? This I believe is what differentiates coaches who run a *great program* versus those who may have a *great team*! The former is based upon the values and leadership of the coach, the latter is based upon the talent of the individual players.

At the professional level, the relationship between coach and player changes. At the professional level everyone is being paid, and the players for the most part are getting paid more than the coaches. So the dynamics are quite different with professional football. It is highly unlikely that Peyton Manning was calling Adam Gase, his quarterback coach with the Denver Broncos, coach. Considering that Peyton is two years older than him and has many more years of experience in playing the game, I would imagine it was more of Adam Gase asking Mr. Manning "what do you think will work here and how do you take your coffee?" That specific relationship, older player, younger coach, is unique to that level of play, and requires a different set of expectations. In this situation, the coach has to earn the player's respect or it simply will not work. It also will require a maturity level of the player to be able to respect someone in a position who may control his destiny, but may have less experience than he does. Even more important, it requires the young coach to demonstrate a confidence to coach a veteran player. That is where the leadership of the head coach and his coordinators become extremely important. Provide that young coach with the confidence and support so that he can be successful.

Is It Important for a Coach to Have Football Playing Experience?

The answer to this is probably pretty easy, and that would be no. There are examples of great coaches in the NFL with no playing experience at all. Presently, going into the 2020 NFL season, 2 head coaches (6.25%) have no football playing experience, 9 coaches signed professional contracts (NFL or CFL), and the remaining 21 coaches played college football. There is an old adage of those who can do, and those who can't teach/coach. There is some truth to that as when you read the biographies of many of the NFL coaches, the stimulus to go into coaching came at the point in their career when they could no longer play. Regardless, their playing experience likely provided some degree of football awareness or instinct. A coach who doesn't have playing experience would have to rely more on calculation and probability than "gut feeling" regarding a decision. Although this may not be a limiting factor, it is likely helpful. Most importantly, the benefit of playing experience, especially in the NFL, is it provides credibility.

When you have been there, it provides a degree of respect for at least one day, your first day. What happens after that is dependent upon the coaches' actions, they can either reinforce the initial impression or lower it, but that is performance and behavior dependent.

When I was hired by the Texas Rangers to serve as a sports science consultant, my responsibilities included educating the players (both major and minor leaguers) on avoiding illegal performance-enhancing drugs, using legal dietary supplements, and assist the strength coach and training staff with issues relating to sport science and training. Jamie Reed, the Director of Sports Medicine for the Rangers, remarked in Senator George Mitchell's report to Major League Baseball that my credibility as a former professional athlete allowed me to easily reach the players and open a two-way dialogue (Mitchell, 2007). I believe that credibility can open an opportunity, but it doesn't guarantee success. There may not have been a NFL head coach with more credibility than Mike Singletary when he became the head coach of the San Francisco 49ers in 2008. He was the leader of one of the most talented defenses that ever was assembled in the NFL with the 1985 Chicago Bears, whose season culminated in a Super Bowl victory. He was an undersized, All-Pro linebacker that defined his position. Despite a high level of credibility, factors for success are quite broad, and Coach Singletary was fired toward the end of the 2010 season. On the other hand, Bill Belichick was a small college football player, with limited credibility as a player. He began his coaching career with the Baltimore Colts in 1975 and slowly worked his way up the coaching ladder. Many consider him as the Greatest Football Coach of All Time, with six Super Bowl victories in nine appearances as a head coach, and another two Super Bowl victories as the defensive coordinator for the New York Giants.

Coaching to the Heart of the Athlete

When I was department chair at the University of Central Florida, the head of our coaching program was Dr. Jeff Duke. Jeff was a football coach at the Florida State University and coached numerous years at the high school level. We talked about coaching for a long time, and one of the things that had really impressed me was his passion for coaching to the heart of the athlete. He was so passionate about this coaching method that he was able to write a book on it, and successfully spread his message on coaching style throughout the country (Duke and Bonham, 2014). His focus of coaching is centered around the player's passion. Have them believe in you as their coach, they will give you everything that they have. To have a player commit 100% to you as a coach and to your program, your message, your passion is one of the true rewards of coaching. If that player trusts that you believe in him and care about him, not just his talent, he will do anything you say. The flip side to that, and it is something I spoke with Dr. Duke about on a number of occasions, is the unfortunate situations where a player realizes that the coach does not care about him, his welfare, or what is in his best interests. It is at that point, that the player, especially at the Division I level, begins thinking "me" versus "we". How does that happen? The player no longer believes that the coach cares. It is not about the x's and o's of the game, it is about the credibility of caring. Do you truly care about the player as a person, without conditions, or do you care about the player who is going to help you get your bonus and your next contract? The players see it, feel it, and show it.

Leadership

If there was one word to describe a head coach, it would be leader. You cannot be a head coach if you do not have leadership skills. You can be an effective football coach but not necessarily a leader. As a coach, you are a teacher and a mentor, but you don't have to be a leader to be effective. However, to be a head coach or a coordinator, leadership skills are imperative. You have to make decisions, speak to the team or unit about game plans, motivate, be able to publicly speak, and represent the team in a professional and dignified manner at all times. Some coaches prefer not to have that responsibility, they are very satisfied as a position coach or perhaps coordinator. They know where their strengths are. Importantly, it doesn't necessarily mean that having those traits as an assistant coach is bad. It actually is good, but you have to make sure to keep your ego in control.

Clash of egos is probably at the route of most internal staff problems. This isn't a football issue, it really is an organizational issue that covers almost every facet of life, whether it be sport, business, academia, or politics. The potential for it increases as the success of individuals within an organization strive to expand their influence and personal growth. Some ego is necessary. If everyone would always agree with what the head coach or group leader wants to do, you have a group of "yes men". This may be much more dangerous than attempting to control ego. Poor leadership and a lack of an alternative thought process may lead your team or organization to step off a cliff. If you have a group of people that follow the leader obediently, without willing to step up and say something when it is necessary, they will and continue to follow that leader off the cliff into oblivion. If the defensive coordinator creates a game plan, and his assistant coaches for some reason all agree, even though there are some obvious flaws and omissions. What needs to be done? If the assistant coach is concerned about hurting the coordinators ego, he needs to find a respectful way to state why the game plan is flawed, and create discussion for an alternative option. In the end, the coordinator and the head coach have the ultimate decision, but coaches comfortable with their knowledge welcome the discussion. It is important for the staff to be on the same page as the game plan is being presented to the players.

One of the more important responsibilities that a coach/leader has is to sell his vision. Communicating his vision in the first meeting to the staff and then to the team is the critical first step. It needs to be done in a straightforward, simple manner that provides a clear and consistent message that is understood by all. To be successful, he has to get the "buy-in" by members of that team. Setting the vision though is not enough. Many leaders can sell a vision or a dream, this is a reflection of their charisma and communication skills, but their job will be dependent on how they go about executing that vision. The most important commodity that any coach/leader has are the folks that work underneath his tutelage. It is important for the leadership to recognize the necessity of teamwork for the organization to achieve success. That has to be the message that is shared. For success to be sustained, the coach has to get the team to share in his vision. Part of that is to make sure that your staff is loyal but provides you with constructive feedback to make any necessary adjustments. Often, one of the most important aspects of your job is hiring the right people.

The hiring process is interesting. As the leader, you have identified certain character traits you expect from your staff. In your contact list, you likely have a number of people that you trust to provide potential recommendations for your coaching staff. You will likely develop a list of potential coaches that you would like to hire before you actually have interviews and make an offer. This is probably the reason why the hiring process of football staff often appear like a coaching merry-go-round, especially at Division I College Football and the NFL. Because these hires are so critical to the team's success, oftentimes coaches don't have the luxury of "taking a chance" on new coaches. Since job security is based upon immediate success, there is some logic for the coach to hire a "known commodity" or someone that he has previous comfort level or has worked with versus the unknown. It is about risk aversion. The rules of minority hiring have attempted to open up dialogue for being more inclusive, whether it has been affective is not clear. However, I do believe that anytime that you put anything but talent and ability as part of any calculus for hiring, the process becomes flawed. The hiring process for coaches is for the most part a completely subjective process, with many of the shortcomings associated with the human element. Without any objective standards, such as education background, experience level, ethics, and integrity, the chance for a "fair" process is minimized. This is where I believe leadership in a number of levels has failed. In an academic institution, especially in Division I college football, it is surprising that college administrators only pay lip service on their demand that coaches be a role model for the student athlete. Why isn't a master's degree in a relevant academic major an appropriate hiring standard? Wouldn't that be a positive effort to enhance student–athlete health and safety? Wouldn't raising minimum academic standards and expectations for coaches help student athletes appreciate the rigor of the coaching position? Coaches would become role models not just for what they say, but also for what they did. Once standards are set, the ability to use inherent prejudices is lowered, not eliminated. Presently, the system is far from being perfect. However, using race as a criterion measure removes the issue of ability from the conversation, and similar to hiring any position in any profession, it should be based upon the most talented individual that brings the most to the table. If college coaches were provided the opportunity to build a program, I believe that the hiring process would be different and opportunities for developing young coaches would improve. If one would look at the lower divisions of football, coaches often become part of the fabric of the university, and are interested and able to build a football program not a football team. Some will move on to work at a more competitive or talented football levels, but others will make a career out of coaching small college football. Regardless, coaches have the ability to impact their players on the values of the game at all levels of play.

Motivation is an important component to all successful coaches. Encouraging and motivating players, as well as their staff, is a critical part of the coach's job, especially during the most difficult parts of a season. Winning is a self-motivating stimulus, but how does a coach motivate a team when they're going through a rough time and have lost several games. A loss in football is not like other sports. You may have a two-week gap between a game. If the last game was lost or you've suffered a few losses, it sits with you for a while. It is not like baseball that can play every day or basketball that plays every couple of days and requires a short memory. This is an on-going battle for a football team. You need to make sure that everyone stays motivated and focused. It is during adverse times where a coach is going to earn his "stripes". It is pretty easy to motivate when things are going well. It is when losses mount that people tend to point fingers and challenge your knowledge. There are also other issues that a coach has to deal with, even when the team is successful. How do you motivate your second string quarterback, or other backup players, who believe that they are good enough to be playing or starting? This is a good problem, because it shows that everyone is working hard to play, but as a coach once your depth chart becomes set, the ability to motivate your players to continue to work hard in practice is critical. You need every player to push each other to stay competitive. You have to make your players believe that hard work will be rewarded, and that the opportunity will eventually present itself. One of the most important lessons in life is exemplified from a quote from Zig Ziglar who remarked that "success occurs when preparation meets opportunity". If that player does not continue to work hard on his skills, when his opportunity comes, he may not be ready. As a coach, you also need to help players set reachable goals. Those small victories help maintain that motivation. One of the hardest players to motivate is upper-level student-athletes who are not part of the regular playing rotation. You need these players to compete in practice, push the starters, and continue to work. However, a player who becomes frustrated because of a lack of playing time may become an issue. The coach has to ensure that it doesn't become a distraction.

When I was coaching at TCNJ, a true freshman player became our starting quarterback. By the time he was a junior, he had lost his starting position to an athlete who was simply better. He was really a good person, worked hard, wanted to compete, and asked if he could come over to the defensive side. The head coach thought it was a good idea, so did the offensive coordinator and he eventually earned playing time in our nickel packages coming up with a couple of big interceptions. Sometimes, the best thing to help a player is perhaps a position change. If a tight end is not playing because he is not as athletic as your other tight ends, would he have a better shot at perhaps moving to the offensive line? Never hesitate to move a player to a position that he can best help the team, and maximize his chances of getting on the field. A second team tight end may make for a very athletic offensive linemen. If you talk with NFL linemen, you may be surprised at how many were skill position players at one point in their youth. Considering how athletic NFL linemen are, this is not surprising.

When football fans think of a coach, they generally picture what he does on game day and practices. He most likely has no idea the amount of hours spent in film review and preparation. Those in the coaching profession understand that well. The fun part of the job is game day. The intensity, the excitement, the competitiveness are all maximized on that day. But to get there requires countless hours of film study and preparation. It can have a significant toll on the family. There is a huge time commitment, especially during the season. You have to watch practice films, game films, and your opponent's game films. However, the coach should insist on efficiency from his staff, and that should trickle down. Most of life is an inverted U. Not enough and you won't be successful, too much and you overtrain or overthink. There is a *sweet spot* that needs to be found that provides the right amount of time, being efficient isn't the opposite of attentive to detail. Too many coaches believe that hours invested equates to wins. Not true, *less is more and more is less*. Coaches, even efficient ones, will spend plenty of time studying film, but the more nights spent sleeping in the office doesn't make you a better team, and it may have you lose the most important team you're on, your family. The coach should be no different than his players in that his health and wellness will go a long way to contributing to his success. The ability to step away and clear your mind actually allows it to declutter, think clearer, and be refreshed. Stress efficiency, you can say how hard you work, but working hard is meaningless unless you are accomplishing something. If you can get the job done in 8 h while others need 10 h, that is efficiency.

Earlier, the discussion of coaching to the heart of the athlete was focused on the player. However, it can easily be applied to your staff. How you treat your staff should be no different than how you treat your players or anyone else for that matter. Coaches also need to be acknowledged for their effort and their contributions appreciated. There have been horror stories of how head football coaches have treated their assistants. One of the most important qualities that a coach can possess is people skills. Your ability to maximize the talent of both your players and coaches will go a long way to achieving success. There is nothing wrong with demanding excellence, but will you do that with a whip or reaching the heart of your staff? If you do the latter, you have a better chance of gaining loyalty and respect. This is where the rubber meets the road in leadership style. It is not just your vision that is critical in setting the framework for success, rather it is also your work ethic, work habits, and how you communicate and treat others that set the tone for how your team will operate. There is nothing more valuable from a leader than their work ethic. Your title will garner initial respect, how you go about your job will sustain, grow, or lose it.

In discussing coaching and leadership, the issues of responsibility and accountability are often forgotten. This has become one of the largest cracks in our society today, and it is not just a football issue. People and organizations tend to justify their actions without taking responsibility or being held accountable. In Chapter 5, an incident that resulted in a number of football players being hospitalized for rhabdomyolysis was discussed. The university where the incident occurred created an investigative committee. Their report did not hold any coach accountable for the hospitalization of those athletes (Drake et al., 2011). Adding insult to injury, the head coach named the strength and conditioning coach, who was responsible for the workout, assistant coach of the year. Although this coach is considered one of the better strength and conditioning coaches in the country today, it does not justify the lack of accountability demonstrated by the football staff and university in brushing under the carpet what had occurred. This was an egregious example of a lack of accountability or responsibility on the part of several university leaders. The fact that no player died was sheer luck.

There have been too many cases of football players dying during spring practice sessions. Universities have paid millions of dollars in settlements, but few have held the head football coach responsible for these negligent events. The only coach to have lost his job as a result of a player's death was D.J. Durkin at the University of Maryland in 2018. It was suggested that the "toxic coaching culture" that Coach Durkin created at the University of Maryland contributed to the death of Jordan McNair (Rittenberg and VanHaaren, 2018). This action made clear that appropriate and safe strength and conditioning programs is part of the responsibility that a coach has toward the health and welfare of his student-athletes. The fact that coaches are more apt to get fired for having a mediocre season than having a player die due to his negligence is all one needs to understand that the system is upside down!

If there was one characteristic that you were to choose in a leader, regardless of whether it is a coach or other position, it would be integrity. A leader with integrity makes the right decision, regardless of the personal consequence or consequence to the team. A leader without integrity, there really isn't anything more that needs to be said. Much of the issues that we see in the world is the direct result of leadership that lacks integrity. We have justified poor behavior in our leadership for many years. Lack of integrity has become more of the norm than a required or expected characteristic. For the sake of our future, we need to demand that integrity is an expectation of leadership, not an exception.

Values of the Game

In the late 1960s and early 1970s, the New York Knicks were actually a great basketball team. They won the NBA championship in 1969 and in 1973. One of stars on those teams was Bill Bradley. He was a Princeton University graduate, and when his playing days were over, he entered politics and became a three-term senator from the state of New Jersey. He eventually was voted into the NBA Hall of Fame, and in 1998 he wrote a book *Values of the Game*. He talked about what he learned from basketball and how he applied it to his life (Bradley, 1998).

Not every athlete understands the value of sport, especially when they are in the middle of playing. Most of the lessons learned are only realized and appreciated when it is over. When the athlete's playing days are over, the transition to a new journey is sometimes very difficult. However, if the player looks back at the values that he was taught as a player, he realizes that the passion, focus, discipline, and work ethic needed to be a successful football player can be applied to other endeavors in life. These traits developed over time as a young athlete never leave, and they simply need to be redressed and applied in a different direction.

Football is one of the few sports where many sacrifice for the glory of someone else. The linemen never get the feel for what it is like to score. It is the success of the team that drives the person. In order for the running back to run across the goal line, for the quarterback to throw the touchdown pass, or the receiver to catch that pass, they need their other ten teammates to do their job. One breakdown will lead to failure. Football is the epitome of teamwork. In most other sports, one player can dominate. Clearly, one player can control the outcome of a basketball game. A pitcher can spend an entire game having a catch with his catcher, the other seven players were spectators. In football, every player has to do his job on every play. You learn to rely on your teammates. The camaraderie developed is what is never forgotten. You feel it as a player, you strive for that as a coach. It is one of the most important values of the game.

Summary

This chapter was different from the other chapters in the book. It was based more on my experiences and beliefs than on the evidence-based approach performed in the previous chapters. Coaching is both a qualitative and quantitative science. Although coaching decisions are often based upon intuition or experience, there are many aspects of the position that require more scientific reasoning. Game plans are based upon the opponent's tendencies. Statistical analysis will help a coach formulate game plans, make checks for specific formations, and help with adjustments. Science also is important as the basis for formulating strength and conditioning programs and player selection and recruitment. However, the responsibility of coaching is more than just the game's tactics. It is also about the responsibility the coach has as a teacher, mentor, and when necessary a father figure. This requires a unique skill set that is exemplified by leadership qualities that can either help or hinder the coach from achieving his goals.

REFERENCES

Abbey EL, Wright CJ, Kirkpatrick CM. Nutrition Practices and Knowledge Among NCAA Division III Football Players. *J Int Soc Sports Nutr*. 14:13, 2017.

Adams J, Bagnall KM, McFadden KD, et al. Body Density Differences Between Negro and Caucasian Professional Football Players. *Br J Sports Med*. 15:257–260, 1981.

Adams WC, Fox RH, Fry AJ, et al. Thermoregulation During Marathon Running in Cold, Moderate and Hot Environments. *J Appl Physiol*. 38:1030–1037, 1975.

Allen TW, Vogel RA, Lincoln AE, et al. Body Size, Body Composition, and Cardiovascular Disease Risk Factors in NFL Players. *Phys Sportsmed*. 38:21–27, 2010.

Alosco ML, Kasimis AB, Stamm JM, et al. Age of First Exposure to American Football and Long-Term Neuropsychiatric and Cognitive Outcomes. *Transl Psychiatry*. 7(9):e1236, 2017a.

Alosco ML, Mez J, Tripodis Y, et al. Age of First Exposure to Tackle Football and Chronic Traumatic Encephalopathy. *Ann Neurol*. 83:886–901, 2018.

Alosco ML, Tripodis Y, Jarnagin J, et al. Repetitive Head Impact Exposure and Later-Life Plasma Total Tau in Former National Football League Players. *Alzheimers Dement (Amst)*. 7:33–40, 2017b.

Alosco ML, Tripodis Y, Rowland B, et al. A Magnetic Resonance Spectroscopy Investigation in Symptomatic Former NFL Players. *Brain Imaging Behav*. doi:10.1007/s11682-019-00060-4, 2019.

American Academy of Sleep Medicine. *The International Classification of Sleep Disorders: Diagnostic and Coding Manual*. 2nd Edition. American Academy of Sleep Medicine, Westchester, IL, 2005.

Anderson S. NCAA Football Off-Season Training: Unanswered Prayers . . . a Prayer Answered. *J Athl Train*. 52:145–148, 2017.

Antonio J, Ellerbroek A, Silver T, et al. The Effects of a High Protein Diet on Indices of Health and Body Composition – a Crossover Trial in Resistance-Trained Men. *J Int Soc Sports Nutr*. 13:3, 2016.

Anzell AR, Potteiger JA, Kraemer WJ, et al. Changes in Height, Body Weight, and Body Composition in American Football Players From 1942 to 2011. *J Strength Cond Res*. 27:277–284, 2013.

Armstrong LE. Research Update: Fluid Replacement and Athlete Hydration. *NSCA J*. 10:69–71, 1988.

Armstrong LE. *Performing in Extreme Environments*. Human Kinetics, Champaign, IL, 2000.

Armstrong LE, Casa DJ, Millard-Stafford M, et al. American College of Sports Medicine Position Stand: Exertional Heat Illness During Training and Competition. *Med Sci Sports Exerc*. 39:556–572, 2007.

Armstrong LE, Johnson EC, Casa DJ, et al. The American Football Uniform: Uncompensable Heat Stress and Hyperthermic Exhaustion. *J Athl Train*. 45:117–127, 2010.

Armstrong LE, Maresh CM. The Induction and Decay of Heat Acclimatization in Trained Athletes. *Sports Med*. 12:302–312, 1991.

Armstrong LE, Maresh CM. The Exertional Heat Illnesses: A Risk of Athletic Participation. *Med Exerc Nutr Health*. 2:125–134, 1993.

Arroyo E, Jajtner AR. Vitamins and Minerals. In Hoffman JR (ed) *Dietary Supplementation in Sport and Exercise*. Routledge, Taylor and Francis Group: Champaign, IL, 22–46, 2019.

Barker M, Wyatt TJ, Johnson RL, et al. Performance Factors, Psychological Assessment, Physical Characteristics, and Football Playing Ability. *J Strength Cond Res*. 7:224–233, 1993.

Barkhoudarian G, Hovda DA, Giza CC. The Molecular Pathophysiology of Concussive Brain Injury – an Update. *Phys Med Rehabil Clin N Am*. 27:373–393, 2016.

Barnes KA, Anderson ML, Stofan JR, et al. Normative Data for Sweating Rate, Sweat Sodium Concentration, and Sweat Sodium Loss in Athletes: An Update and Analysis by Sport. *J Sports Sci*. 37:2356–2366, 2019.

Baron SL, Hein MJ, Lehman E, et al. Body Mass Index, Playing Position, Race, and the Cardiovascular Mortality of Retired Professional Football Players. *Am J Cardiol*. 109:889–896, 2012.

Basser PJ, Pierpaoli C. Microstructural and Physiological Features of Tissues Elucidated by Quantitative-Diffusion-Tensor MRI. *J Magn Reson. B*. 111:209–219, 1996.

Bayliff GE, Jacobson BH, Moghaddam M, et al. Global Positioning System Monitoring of Selected Physical Demands of NCAA Division I Football Players During Games. *J Strength Cond Res*. 33:1185–1191, 2019.

Beaulieu-Jones BR, Rossy WH, Sanchez G, et al. Epidemiology of Injuries Identified at the NFL Scouting Combine and Their Impact on Performance in the National Football League: Evaluation of 2203 Athletes From 2009 to 2015. *Orthop J Sports Med*. 5(7). doi:10.1177/2325967117708744, 2017.

Bemben MG, Bemben DA, Loftiss DD, et al. Creatine Supplementation During Resistance Training in College Football Athletes. *Med Sci Sports Exerc*. 33:1667–1673, 2001.

Berg K, Latin RW, Baechle T. Physical and Performance Characteristics of NCAA Division I Football Players. *Res Quart*. 61:395–401, 1990.

Bergh U, Ekblom B. Influence of Muscle Temperature on Maximal Muscle Strength and Power Output in Human Muscle. *Acta Physiol Scand*. 107:332–337, 1979.

Bergstrom J, Hermansen L, Hultman E, et al. Diet, Muscle Glycogen and Physical Performance. *Acta Physiol Scand*. 71:140–150, 1967.

Bjorntorp P. Importance of Fat as a Support Nutrient for Energy: Metabolism of Athletes. *J Sports Sci*. 9:71–76, 1991.

Black W, Roundy E. Comparisons of Size, Strength, Speed and Power in NCAA Division I-A Football Players. *J Strength Cond Res*. 8:80–85, 1994.

Bohner JD, Hoffman JR, McCormack WP, et al. Moderate Altitude Affects High Intensity Running Performance in a Collegiate Women's Soccer Game. *J Hum Kinet*. 47:147–154, 2015.

Boirie Y, Dangin M, Gachon P, et al. Slow and Fast Dietary Proteins Differently Modulate Postprandial Protein Accretion. *Proc Nat Acad Sci*. 94:14930–14935, 1997.

Boldyrev A, Bulygina E, Leinsoo T, et al. Protection of Neuronal Cells Against Reactive Oxygen Species by Carnosine and Related Compounds. *Comp Biochem Physiol Part B: Biochem Mol Biol*. 137:81–88, 2004.

Boldyrev A, Stvolinsky S, Fedorova T, et al. Carnosine as a Natural Antioxidant and Geroprotector: From Molecular Mechanisms to Clinical Trials. *Rej Res*. 13:156–158, 2010.

Bosch TA, Burruss TP, Weir NL, et al. Abdominal Body Composition Differences in NFL Football Players. *J Strength Cond Res*. 28:3313–3319, 2014.

Bosch TA, Carbuhn AF, Stanforth PR, et al. Body Composition and Bone Mineral Density of Division 1 Collegiate Football Players: A Consortium of College Athlete Research Study. *J Strength Cond Res*. 33:1339–1346, 2019.

Bradley B. *Values of the Game*. Artisan Books: New York, NY, 1998.

Brajkovic D, Ducharme MB. Finger Dexterity, Skin Temperature, and Blood Flow During Auxiliary Heating in the Cold. *J Appl Physiol*. 95:758–770, 2003.

Burke LM, Collier GR, Hargreaves M. Glycemic Index – A New Tool in Sport Nutrition? *Int J Sport Nutr*. 8:401–415, 1998.

Casa DJ, Anderson SA, Baker L, et al. The Inter-Association Task Force for Preventing Sudden Death in Collegiate Conditioning Sessions: Best Practices Recommendations. *J Athl Train*. 47:477–480, 2012.

Casson IR, Viano DC, Powell JW, et al. Twelve Years of National Football League Concussion Data. *Sports Health*. 2:471–483, 2010.

Caswell SV, Ausborn A, Diao G, et al. Anthropometrics, Physical Performance, and Injury Characteristics of Youth American Football. *Orthop J Sports Med*. 4(8). doi:10.1177/2325967116662251, 2016.

Chang AY, FitzGerald SJ, Cannaday J, et al. Cardiovascular Risk Factors and Coronary Atherosclerosis in Retired National Football League Players. *Am J Cardiol*. 104:805–811, 2009.

Channell BT, Barfield JP. Effect of Olympic and Traditional Resistance Training on Vertical Jump Improvement in High School Boys. *J Strength Cond Res*. 22:1522–1527, 2008.

Chen Y, Herrold AA, Gallagher VT, et al. Cutting to the Pathophysiology Chase: Translating Cutting-Edge Neuroscience to Rehabilitation Practice in Sports-Related Concussion Management. *J Orthop Sports Phys Ther*. 49:811–818, 2019.

Cheung SS. *Advanced Environmental Exercise Physiology*. Human Kinetics Publishers: Champaign, IL, 2009.

Claremont AD, Nagle F, Reddan WD, et al. Comparison of Metabolic, Temperature, Heart Rate and Ventilatory Responses to Exercise at Extreme Ambient Temperatures (0° and 35°C). *Med Sci Sport Exerc*. 7:150–154, 1975.

Clark MD, Asken BM, Marshall SW, et al. Descriptive Characteristics of Concussions in National Football League Games, 2010–2011 to 2013–2014. *Am J Sports Med*. 45:929–936, 2017.

Clark MD, Varangis EML, Champagne AA, et al. Effects of Career Duration, Concussion History, and Playing Position on White Matter Microstructure and Functional Neural Recruitment in Former College and Professional Football Athletes. *Radiology*. 286:976–977, 2018.

Cole CR, Salvaterra GF, Davis JE Jr, et al. Evaluation of Dietary Practices of National Collegiate Athletic Association Division I Football Players. *J Strength Cond Res*. 19:490–494, 2005.

Connolly JG, Nathanson JT, Sobotka S, et al. Effect of Playing and Training at Altitude on Concussion Incidence in Professional Football. *Orthop J Sports Med*. 6(12). doi:10.1177/2325967118794928, 2018.

Connor J, Woolf J, Mazanov J. Would They Dope? Revisiting the Goldman Dilemma. *Br J Sports Med*. 47:697–700, 2013.

Cooper ER, Ferrara MS, Casa DJ, et al. Exertional Heat Illness in American Football Players: When Is the Risk Greatest? *J Athl Train*. 51:593–600, 2016.

Costill DL. Carbohydrates for Exercise: Dietary Demands for Optimal Performance. *Int J Sports Med*. 9:1–18, 1988.

Crabtree-Hannigan J. *Dabo Swinney, Nick Saban and the 10 Highest-Paid College Football Coaches in 2019*, 2020. www.sportingnews.com/us/ncaa-football/news/highest-paid-college-football-coaches-2019-dabo-swinney-nick-saban/1tm0hym5dtina1ms02d4davsfp.

Craig C, Overbeek RW, Condon MV, et al. A Relationship Between Temperature and Aggression in NFL Football Penalties. *J Sport Health Sci*. 5:205–210, 2016.

Crouse SF, White S, Erwin JP, et al. Echocardiographic and Blood Pressure Characteristics of First-Year Collegiate American-Style Football Players. *Am J Cardiol*. 117:131–134, 2016.

Davies CTM, Mecrow IK, White MJ. Contractile Properties of the Human Triceps Surae With Some Observations on the Effects of Temperature and Exercise. *Eur J Appl Physiol*. 49:255–269, 1982.

Davies CTM, Young K. Effects of Training at 30 and 100% Maximal Isometric Force on the Contractile Properties of the Triceps Surae of Man. *J Physiol*. 336:22–23, 1983.

DeMartini-Nolan JK, Martschinske JL, Casa D, et al. Physical Demands of National Collegiate Athletic Association Division I Football Players During Preseason Training in the Heat. *J Strength Cond Res*. 25:2935–2943, 2011.

DeMartini-Nolan JK, Martschinske JL, Casa DJ, et al. Examining the Influence of Exercise Intensity and Hydration on Gastrointestinal Temperature in Collegiate Football Players. *J Strength Cond Res*. 32:2888–2896, 2018.

Dengel DR, Bosch TA, Burruss TP, et al. Body Composition and Bone Mineral Density of National Football League Players. *J Strength Cond Res*. 28:1–6, 2014.

Dick R, Agel J, Marshall SW. National Collegiate Athletic Association Injury Surveillance System Commentaries: Introduction and Methods. *J Athl Train*. 42:173–182, 2007a.

Dick R, Ferrara MS, Agel J, et al. Descriptive Epidemiology of Collegiate Men's Football Injuries: National Collegiate Athletic Association Injury Surveillance System, 1988–1989 Through 2003–2004. *J Athl Train*. 42:221–233, 2007b.

Dienstbier RA. Behavioral Correlates of Sympathoadrenal Reactivity: The Toughness Model. *Med Sci Sports Exerc*. 23:846–852, 1991.

Dompier TP, Kerr ZY, Marshall SW, et al. Incidence of Concussion During Practice and Games in Youth, High School, and Collegiate American Football Players. *JAMA Pediatr.* 169:659–665, 2015.

Drake DR, Herwaldt L, Hines NW, et al. *Report of the Special Presidential Committee to Investigate the January 2011 Hospitalization of University of Iowa Football Players.* University Report, March 21, 2011.

Duke J, Bonham C. *3D Coach: Capturing the Heart Behind the Jersey.* Baker Publishing Group: Ada, MI, 2014.

Dupler TL, Amonette WE, Coleman AE, et al. Anthropometric and Performance Differences Among High-School Football Players. *J Strength Cond Res.* 24:1975–1982, 2010.

Edenfield KM, Reifsteck F, Carek S, et al. Echocardiographic Measurements of Left Ventricular End-Diastolic Diameter and Interventricular Septal Diameter in Collegiate Football Athletes at Preparticipation Evaluation Referenced to Body Surface Area. *BMJ Open Sport Exerc Med.* 5:e000488, 2019.

Ehlers GG, Ball TE, Liston L. Creatine Kinase Levels Are Elevated During 2-A-Day Practices in Collegiate Football Players. *J Athl Train.* 37:151–156, 2002.

Eley HL, Russell ST, Baxter JH, et al. Signaling Pathways Initiated by Beta-Hydroxy-Beta-Methylbutyrate to Attenuate the Depression of Protein Synthesis in Skeletal Muscle in Response to Cachectic Stimuli. *Am J Physiol Endocr Metab.* 293:E923–E931, 2007.

Elliot TA, Cree MG, Sanford AP, et al. Milk Ingestion Stimulates Net Muscle Protein Synthesis Following Resistance Exercise. *Med Sci Sports Exerc.* 38:667–674, 2006.

Elliott KR, Harmatz JS, Zhao Y, et al. Body Size Changes Among National Collegiate Athletic Association New England Division III Football Players, 1956–2014: Comparison With Age-Matched Population Controls. *J Athl Train.* 51:373–381, 2016.

Epstein Y. Heat Intolerance: Predisposing Factor or Residual Injury. *Med Sci Sports Exerc.* 22:29–35, 1990.

Ferguson, Daniel David Reid. *Utilizing Analytics in American Football to Improve Decision Making on Fourth Down.* Graduate Theses, Engineering Management 7, 2018. https://scholar.rose-hulman.edu/engineering_management_grad_theses/7.

Ferretti G. Cold and Muscle Performance. *Int J Sports Med.* 13(supp):S185–S187, 1992.

Fitzgerald CF, Jensen RL. A Comparison of the National Football League's Annual National Football League Combine 1999–2000 to 2015–2016. *J Strength Cond Res.* 34:771–781, 2020.

Flatt AA, Esco MR, Allen JR, et al. Heart Rate Variability and Training Load Among National Collegiate Athletic Association Division 1 College Football Players Throughout Spring Camp. *J Strength Cond Res.* 32:3127–3134, 2018.

Fry AC, Kraemer WJ. Physical Performance Characteristics of American Collegiate Football Players. *J Appl Sport Sci Res.* 5:126–138, 1991.

Funk JR, Rowson S, Daniel RW, et al. Validation of Concussion Risk Curves for Collegiate Football Players Derived From HITS Data. *Ann Biomed Eng.* 40:79–89, 2012.

Garstecki MA, Latin RW, Cuppett MM. Comparison of Selected Physical Fitness and Performance Variables Between NCAA Division I and II Football Players. *J Strength Cond Res.* 18:292–297, 2004.

Ge RL, Witkowski S, Zhang Y, et al. Determinants of Erythropoietin Release in Response to Short-Term Hypobaric Hypoxia. *J Appl Physiol.* 92:2361–2367, 2002.

Gepner Y, Varanoske AN, Boffey D, et al. Benefits of HMB Supplementation in Trained and Untrained Individuals. *Res Sports Med.* 27:204–218, 2019.

Gill J, Merchant-Borna K, Jeromin A, et al. Acute Plasma Tau Relates to Prolonged Return to Play After Concussion. *Neurology.* 88:595–602, 2017.

Givoni B, Goldman RF. Predicting Rectal Temperature Response to Work, Environment, and Clothing. *J Appl Physiol.* 21:812–822, 1972.

Giza CC, Hovda DA. The New Neurometabolic Cascade of Concussion. *Neurosurgery.* 75(supp 4):S24–S33, 2014.

Godek SF, Bartolozzi AR, Burkholder R, et al. Sweat Rates and Fluid Turnover in Professional Football Players: A Comparison of National Football League Linemen and Backs. *J Athl Train.* 43:184–189, 2008.

Godek SF, Godek JJ, Bartolozzi AR. Hydration Status in College Football Players During Consecutive Days of Twice-a-Day Preseason Practices. *Am J Sports Med.* 33:843–851, 2005.

Godt RE, Lindly BD. Influence of Temperature Upon Contractile Activation and Isometric Force Production in Mechanically Skinned Muscle Fibers of the Frog. *J Gen Physiol.* 80:279–297, 1982.

Goldman B, Bush PJ, Klatz R. *Death in the Locker Room*. Century: London, 32, 1984.

Golightly YM, Marshall SW, Callahan LF, et al. Early-Onset Arthritis in Retired National Football League Players. *J Phys Act Health*. 6:638–643, 2009.

Gomes EC, Silva AN, Oliveira MR. Oxidants, Antioxidants, and the Beneficial Roles of Exercise-Induced Production of Reactive Species. *Oxid Med Cell Longev*. 2012:1–12, 2012.

Goswami R, Dufort P, Tartaglia MC, et al. Frontotemporal Correlates of Impulsivity and Machine Learning in Retired Professional Athletes With a History of Multiple Concussions. *Brain Struct Funct*. 221:1911–1925, 2016.

Grashow R, Weisskopf MG, Miller KK, et al. Association of Concussion Symptoms With Testosterone Levels and Erectile Dysfunction in Former Professional US-Style Football Players. *JAMA Neurol*. 76:1428–1438, 2019.

Grundstein AJ, Hosokawa Y, Casa DJ. Fatal Exertional Heat Stroke and American Football Players: The Need for Regional Heat-Safety Guidelines. *J Athl Train*. 53:43–50, 2018.

Grundstein AJ, Knox JA, Vanos J, et al. American Football and Fatal Exertional Heat Stroke: A Case Study of Korey Stringer. *Int J Biometeorol*. 61:1471–1480, 2017.

Guskiewicz KM, Marshall SW, Bailes J, et al. Association Between Recurrent Concussion and Late-Life Cognitive Impairment in Retired Professional Football Players. *Neurosurgery*. 57:719–726, 2005.

Guskiewicz KM, Marshall SW, Bailes J, et al. Recurrent Concussion and Risk of Depression in Retired Professional Football Players. *Med Sci Sports Exerc*. 39:903–909, 2007.

Guskiewicz KM, McCrea M, Marshall SW, et al. Cumulative Effects Associated With Recurrent Concussion in Collegiate Football Players: The NCAA Concussion Study. *JAMA*. 290:2549–2555, 2003.

Guskiewicz KM, Weaver NL, Padua DA, et al. Epidemiology of Concussion in Collegiate and High School Football Players. *Am J Sports Med*. 28:643–650, 2000.

Gwacham N, Wagner DR. Acute Effects of a Caffeine-Taurine Energy Drink on Repeated Sprint Performance of American College Football Players. *Int J Sport Nutr Exerc Metab*. 22:109–116, 2012.

Haff GC, Whitley A, Potteiger JA. A Brief Review: Explosive Exercises in Sports Performance. *Strength Cond J*. 23:13–20, 2001.

Hamlin MJ, Hinckson EA, Wood MR, et al. Simulated Rugby Performance at 1550-m Altitude Following Adaptation to Intermittent Normobaric Hypoxia. *J Sci Med Sport*. 11:593–599, 2008.

Harmon KG, Drezner JA, Gammons M, et al. American Medical Society for Sports Medicine Position Statement: Concussion in Sport. *Br J Sports Med*. 47:15–26, 2013.

Harris RC, Tallon MJ, Dunnett M, et al. The Absorption of Orally Supplied β-Alanine and Its Effect on Muscle Carnosine Synthesis in Human Vastus Lateralis. *Amino Acids*. 30:279–289, 2006.

Hart J Jr, Kraut MA, Womack KB, et al. Neuroimaging of Cognitive Dysfunction and Depression in Aging Retired National Football League Players: A Cross-Sectional Study. *JAMA Neurol*. 70:326–335, 2013.

Havenith G, Holmér I, den Hartog EA, et al. Clothing Evaporative Heat Resistance – Proposal for Improved Representation in Standards and Models. *Ann Occup Hyg*. 43:339–346, 1999.

Hershman EB, Anderson R, Bergfeld JA, et al. National Football League Injury and Safety Panel: An Analysis of Specific Lower Extremity Injury Rates on Grass and FieldTurf Playing Surfaces in National Football League Games: 2000–2009 Seasons. *Am J Sports Med*. 40:2200–2205, 2012.

Heus R, Daanen HAM, Havenith G. Physiological Criteria for Functioning of Hands in the Cold. *Appl Ergon*. 26:5–13, 1995.

Hiskens MI, Schneiders AG, Angoa-Pérez M, et al. Blood Biomarkers for Assessment of Mild Traumatic Brain Injury and Chronic Traumatic Encephalopathy. *Biomarkers*. 2020:1–15, 2020 [published online ahead of print, March 12, 2020].

Hitchcock KM, Millard-Stafford ML, Phillips JM, et al. Metabolic and Thermoregulatory Responses to a Simulated American Football Practice in the Heat. *J Strength Cond Res*. 21:710–717, 2007.

Hoffman JR. Endocrinology of Sport Competition. In Kraemer WJ, Rogol AD (eds) *The Endocrinology of Physical Exercise and Sport*. Blackwell Publishing: Oxford, England, 600–612, 2005.

Hoffman JR. The Applied Physiology of American Football. *Int J Sport Physiol Perf*. 3:387–392, 2008.

Hoffman JR. *Physiological Aspects of Sport Training and Performance*. 2nd Edition. Human Kinetics: Champaign, IL, 2014.

Hoffman JR. Physiological Demands of American Football. *Gatorade Sports Sci Exchange*. 28(143):1–6, 2015.

Hoffman JR. Dietary Supplementation: Prevalence of Use, Regulation and Safety. In Hoffman JR (ed) *Dietary Supplementation in Sport and Exercise*. Routledge, Taylor and Francis Group: New York, NY, 1–21, 2019a.

Hoffman JR. Energy Drinks. In Hoffman JR (ed) *Dietary Supplementation in Sport and Exercise*. Routledge, Taylor and Francis Group: New York, NY, 233–246, 2019b.

Hoffman JR, Cooper J, Wendell M, et al. Comparison of Olympic Versus Traditional Power Lifting Training Programs in Football Players. *J Strength Cond Res*. 18:129–135, 2004a.

Hoffman JR, Cooper J, Wendell M, et al. Effects of Beta-Hydroxy Beta-Methylbutyrate on Power Performance and Indices of Muscle Damage and Stress During High-Intensity Training. *J Strength Cond Res*. 18:747–752, 2004b.

Hoffman JR, Faigenbaum AD, Ratamess NA, et al. Nutritional Supplementation and Anabolic Steroid Use in Adolescents. *Med Sci Sports Exerc*. 40:15–24, 2008a.

Hoffman JR, Falvo MJ. Protein – Which Is Best? *J Sports Sci Med*. 3:118–130, 2004d.

Hoffman JR, Fry AC, Deschenes M, Kemp M, Kraemer WJ. The Effects of Self-Selection for Frequency of Training in a Winter Conditioning Program or Football. *J Applied Sport Sci Res*. 4:76–82, 1990.

Hoffman JR, Hamilton E. Wall-Mounted Sled Training and Testing for Football Players. *Strength Cond J*. 24:9–13, 2002.

Hoffman JR, Im J, Kang J, et al. The Effect of a Competitive Collegiate Football Season on Power Performance and Muscle Oxygen Recovery Kinetics. *J Strength Cond Res*. 19:509–513, 2004c.

Hoffman JR, Kang J. Strength Changes During an Inseason Resistance Training Program for Football. *J Strength Cond Res*. 17:109–114, 2003.

Hoffman JR, Kang J, Ratamess NA, et al. Biochemical and Hormonal Responses During an Intercollegiate Football Season. *Med Sci Sports Exerc*. 37:1237–1241, 2005a.

Hoffman JR, Kraemer WJ, Bhasin S, et al. Position Stand on Androgen and Human Growth Hormone Use. *J Strength Cond Res*. 23(supp 5):S1–S59, 2009c.

Hoffman JR, Maresh CM, Newton RU, et al. Performance, Biochemical, and Endocrine Changes During a Competitive American Football Game. *Med Sci Sports Exerc*. 34:1845–1853, 2002.

Hoffman JR, Ratamess NA, Cooper JJ, et al. Comparison of Loaded and Unloaded Jump Squat Training on Strength/Power Performance in College Football Players. *J Strength Cond Res*. 19:810–815, 2005b.

Hoffman JR, Ratamess NA, Faigenbaum AD, et al. Short-Duration Beta-Alanine Supplementation Increases Training Volume and Reduces Subjective Feelings of Fatigue in College Football Players. *Nutr Res*. 28:31–35, 2008b.

Hoffman JR, Ratamess NA, Kang J. Performance Changes During a College Playing Career in NCAA Division III Football Athletes. *J Strength Cond Res*. 25:2351–2357, 2011.

Hoffman JR, Ratamess NA, Kang J, et al. Effect of Creatine and Beta-Alanine Supplementation on Performance and Endocrine Responses in Strength/Power Athletes. *Int J Sport Nutr Exerc Metab*. 16:430–446, 2006a.

Hoffman JR, Ratamess NA, Kang J, et al. Effects of Protein Intake on Strength, Body Composition and Endocrine Changes in Strength/Power Athletes. *J Int Soc Sports Nutr*. 3:12–18, 2006b.

Hoffman JR, Ratamess NA, Kang J, et al. Effects of Protein Supplementation on Muscular Performance and Resting Hormonal Changes in College Football Players. *J Sports Sci Med*. 6:85–92, 2007.

Hoffman JR, Ratamess NA, Klatt M, et al. Comparison Between Different Resistance Training Programs in Division III American College Football Players. *J Strength Cond Res*. 23:11–19, 2009a.

Hoffman JR, Ratamess NA, Tranchina CP, et al. Effect of Protein Supplement Timing on Strength, Power and Body Compositional Changes in Resistance-Trained Men. *Int J Sport Nutr Exerc Metab*. 19:172–185, 2009b.

Hoffman JR, Ratamess NA, Tranchina CP, et al. Effect of Protein Ingestion on Recovery Indices Following a Resistance Training Protocol in Strength/Power Athletes. *Amino Acids*. 38:771–778, 2010.

Hoffman JR, Stavsky H, Falk B. The Effect of Water Restriction on Anaerobic Power and Vertical Jumping Height in Basketball Players. *Int J Sports Med*. 16:214–218, 1995.

Hoffman JR, Tenenbaum G, Maresh CM, et al. Relationship Between Athletic Performance Tests and Playing Time in Elite College Basketball Players. *J Strength Cond Res*. 10:67–71, 1996.

Hoffman JR, Varanoske AN, Stout JR. Effects of β-Alanine Supplementation on Carnosine Elevation and Physiological Performance. *Advances in Food and Nutrition Research*. 84:183–206, 2018.

Hoffman JR, Wendell M, Cooper J, et al. Comparison Between Linear and Nonlinear In-Season Training Programs in Freshman Football Players. *J Strength Cond Res.* 17:561–565, 2003.

Hoffman JR, Williams DR, Emerson NS, et al. L-Alanyl-L-Glutamine Ingestion Maintains Performance During a Competitive Basketball Game. *J Int Soc Sports Nutr.* 9:4, 2012.

Honig A. Role of Arterial Chemoreceptors in the Reflex Control of Renal Function and Body Fluid Volumes in Acute Arterial Hypoxia. In Acher H, O'Regan RG (eds) *Physiology of the Peripheral Arterial Chemoreceptors.* Elsevier: Amsterdam, 395–429, 1983.

Horn S, Gregory P, Guskiewicz KM. Self-Reported Anabolic-Androgenic Steroids Use and Musculoskeletal Injuries: Findings From the Center for the Study of Retired Athletes Health Survey of Retired NFL Players. *Am J Phys Med Rehabil.* 88:192–200, 2009.

Horswill CA, Hickner RC, Scott JR, et al. Weight Loss, Dietary Carbohydrate Modifications and High Intensity Physical Performance. *Med Sci Sports Exerc.* 22:470–476, 1990.

Howard RL, Kraemer WJ, Stanley DC, et al. The Effects of Cold Immersion on Muscle Strength. *J Strength Cond Res.* 8:129–133, 1994.

Iosia MF, Bishop PA. Analysis of Exercise-to-Rest Ratios During Division IA Televised Football Competition. *J Strength Cond Res.* 22:332–340, 2008.

Irick E. *Student-Athlete Participation 1981-82-2018-19: NCAA® Sports Sponsorship and Participation Rates Report*, 2019. https://ncaaorg.s3.amazonaws.com/research/sportpart/2018-19RES_SportsSponsorship ParticipationRatesReport.pdf. Accessed March 28, 2020.

Issurin VB. Benefits and Limitations of Block Periodized Training Approaches to Athletes' Preparation: A Review. *Sports Med.* 46:329–338, 2016.

Ivy JL, Katz AL, Cutler CL, et al. Muscle Glycogen Synthesis After Exercise: Effect of Time of Carbohydrate Ingestion. *J Appl Physiol.* 64:1480–1485, 1988.

Jacobson BH, Conchola EG, Glass RG, et al. Longitudinal Morphological and Performance Profiles for American, NCAA Division I Football Players. *J Strength Cond Res.* 27:2347–2354, 2013.

Jäger R, Kerksick CM, Campbell BI, et al. International Society of Sports Nutrition Position Stand: Protein and Exercise. *J Int Soc Sports Nutr.* 14:20, 2017.

Janssen PH, Mandrekar J, Mielke MM, et al. High School Football and Late-Life Risk of Neurodegenerative Syndromes, 1956–1970. *Mayo Clin Proc.* 92:66–71, 2017.

Jehue R, Street D, Huizenga R. Effect of Time Zone and Game Time Changes on Team Performance: National Football League. *Med Sci Sports Exerc.* 25:127–131, 1993.

Johnson EC, Ganio MS, Lee EC, et al. Perceptual Responses While Wearing an American Football Uniform in the Heat. *J Athl Train.* 45:107–116, 2010.

Johnson W. *Steroids: A Problem of Huge Dimensions.* Sports Illustrated, May 13, 1985. https://vault.si.com/vault/1985/05/13/steroids-a-problem-of-huge-dimensions. Accessed April 16, 2020.

Judge LW, Kumley RF, Bellar DM, et al. Hydration and Fluid Replacement Knowledge, Attitudes, Barriers, and Behaviors of NCAA Division 1 American Football Players. *J Strength Cond Res.* 30:2972–2978, 2016.

Judge LW, Petersen JC, Bellar DM, et al. The Current State of NCAA Division I Collegiate Strength Facilities: Size, Equipment, Budget, Staffing, and Football Status. *J Strength Cond Res.* 28:2253–2261, 2014.

Kelly DF, Chaloner C, Evans D, et al. Prevalence of Pituitary Hormone Dysfunction, Metabolic Syndrome, and Impaired Quality of Life in Retired Professional Football Players: A Prospective Study. *J Neurotrauma.* 31:1161–1171, 2014.

Kenefick RW, Cheuvront SN, Castellani JW, et al. Thermal Stress. In Davis JR, Johnson R, Stepanek J, Fogarty JA (eds) *Fundamentals of Aerospace Medicine*, 4th Edition. Wolter Kluwer, Lippincott Williams and Wilkins: Philadelphia, PA, 206–220, 2008.

Kerksick CM, Arent S, Schoenfeld BJ, et al. International Society of Sports Nutrition Position Stand: Nutrient Timing. *J Int Soc Sports Nutr.* 14:33, 2017.

Kern BD, Robinson TL. Effects of β-Alanine Supplementation on Performance and Body Composition in Collegiate Wrestlers and Football Players. *J Strength Cond Res.* 25:1804–1815, 2011.

Kerr ZY, Marshall SW, Dompier TP, et al. College Sports-Related Injuries – United States, 2009–10 Through 2013–14 Academic Years. *MMWR Morb Mortal Wkly Rep.* 64:1330–1336, 2015.

Kerr ZY, Marshall SW, Harding HP Jr, et al. Nine-Year Risk of Depression Diagnosis Increases With Increasing Self-Reported Concussions in Retired Professional Football Players. *Am J Sports Med.* 40:2206–2212, 2012.

Kerr ZY, Register-Mihalik JK, Pryor RR, et al. The Association Between Mandated Preseason Heat Acclimatization Guidelines and Exertional Heat Illness During Preseason High School American Football Practices. *Environ Health Perspect.* 127:47003, 2019.

Kerr ZY, Simon JE, Grooms DR, et al. Epidemiology of Football Injuries in the National Collegiate Athletic Association, 2004–2005 to 2008–2009. *Orthop J Sports Med.* 4(9). doi:10.1177/2325967116664500, 2016a.

Kerr ZY, Wilkerson GB, Caswell SV, et al. The First Decade of Web-Based Sports Injury Surveillance: Descriptive Epidemiology of Injuries in United States High School Football (2005–2006 Through 2013–2014) and National Collegiate Athletic Association Football (2004–2005 Through 2013–2014). *J Athl Train.* 53:738–751, 2018.

Kerr ZY, Yeargin SW, Hosokawa Y, et al. The Epidemiology and Management of Exertional Heat Illnesses in High School Sports During the 2012/2013–2016/2017 Academic Years. *J Sport Rehabil.* 6:1–7, 2019.

Kerr ZY, Zuckerman SL, Wasserman EB, et al. Concussion Symptoms and Return to Play Time in Youth, High School, and College American Football Athletes. *JAMA Pediatr.* 170:647–653, 2016b.

Kim JH, Hollowed C, Patel K, et al. Temporal Changes in Cardiovascular Remodeling Associated With Football Participation. *Med Sci Sports Exerc.* 50:1892–1898, 2018.

Kirwan RD, Kordick LK, McFarland S, et al. Dietary, Anthropometric, Blood-Lipid, and Performance Patterns of American College Football Players During 8 Weeks of Training. *Int J Sport Nutr Exerc Metab.* 22:444–451, 2012.

Klein C. *How Teddy Roosevelt Saved Football,* 2012. www.history.com/news/how-teddy-roosevelt-saved-football. Accessed April 1, 2020.

Kohen R, Yamamoto Y, Cundy KC, et al. Antioxidant Activity of Carnosine, Homocarnosine, and Anserine Present in Muscle and Brain. *Proc Nat Acad Sci.* 85:3175–3179, 1988.

Kraemer WJ, Gotshalk LA. Physiology of American Football. In Garrett WE, Kirkendall DT (eds) *Exercise and Sport Science.* Lippincott Williams and Wilkins: Philadelphia, PA, 795–813, 2000.

Kraemer WJ, Hooper DR, Kupchak BR, et al. The Effects of a Roundtrip Trans-American Jet Travel on Physiological Stress, Neuromuscular Performance, and Recovery. *J Appl Physiol.* 121:438–448, 2016.

Kraemer WJ, Looney DP, Martin GJ, et al. Changes in Creatine Kinase and Cortisol in National Collegiate Athletic Association Division I American Football Players During a Season. *J Strength Cond Res.* 27:434–441, 2013.

Kraemer WJ, Newton RU. Training for Muscular Power. *Phys Med Rehab Clin.* 11:341–367, 2000.

Kraemer WJ, Spiering BA, Volek JS, et al. Recovery From a National Collegiate Athletic Association Division I Football Game: Muscle Damage and Hormonal Status. *J Strength Cond Res.* 23:2–10, 2009.

Kraemer WJ, Torine JC, Silvestre R, et al. Body Size and Composition of National Football League Players. *J Strength Cond Res.* 19:485–489, 2005.

Kreider RB, Ferreira M, Greenwood M, et al. Effects of Calcium β-HMB Supplementation During Training on Markers of Catabolism, Body Composition, Strength and Sprint Performance. *JEP Online.* 3:48–59, 2000.

Kreider RB, Ferreira M, Wilson M, et al. Effects of Creatine Supplementation on Body Composition, Strength, and Sprint Performance. *Med Sci Sports Exerc.* 30:73–82, 1998.

Kucera KL, Klossner D, Colgate B, et al. *Annual Survey of Football Injury Research 1931–2016.* National Center for Catastrophic Sports Injury Research: Chapel Hill, NC, 2017. Accessed April 7, 2020.

Kumar NS, Chin M, O'Neill C, et al. On-Field Performance of National Football League Players After Return From Concussion. *Am J Sports Med.* 42:2050–2055, 2014.

Kupchak BR, Kraemer WJ, Hooper DR, et al. The Effects of a Transcontinental Flight on Markers of Coagulation and Fibrinolysis in Healthy Men After Vigorous Physical Activity. *Chronobiol Int.* 34:148–161, 2017.

Kuzmits FE, Adams AJ. The NFL Combine: Does It Predict Performance in the National Football League? *J Strength Cond Res.* 22:1721–1727, 2008.

Laskas JM, Veasay N. Bennet Omalu, Concussions, and the NFL: How One Doctor Changed Football Forever. *GQ Magazine,* 2009.

Lawrence DW, Comper P, Hutchison MG. Influence of Extrinsic Risk Factors on National Football League Injury Rates. *Orthop J Sports Med.* 4. doi:10.1177/2325967116639222, 2016.

Lawrence DW, Hutchison MG, Comper P. Descriptive Epidemiology of Musculoskeletal Injuries and Concussions in the National Football League, 2012–2014. *Orthop J Sports Med.* 3(5). doi:10.1177/2325967115583653, 2015.

Lehman EJ, Hein MJ, Baron SL, et al. Neurodegenerative Causes of Death Among Retired National Football League Players. *Neurology.* 79:1970–1974, 2012.

Lepage C, Muehlmann M, Tripodis Y, et al. Limbic System Structure Volumes and Associated Neurocognitive Functioning in Former NFL Players. *Brain Imaging Behav.* 13:725–734, 2019.

Leutzinger TJ, Gillen ZM, Miramonti AM, et al. Anthropometric and Athletic Performance Combine Test Results Among Positions Within Grade Levels of High School-Aged American Football Players. *J Strength Cond Res.* 32:1288–1296, 2018.

Lin A, Charney M, Shenton ME, et al. Chronic Traumatic Encephalopathy: Neuroimaging Biomarkers. *Handb Clin Neurol.* 158:309–322, 2018.

Lin J, Wang F, Weiner RB, et al. Blood Pressure and LV Remodeling Among American-Style Football Players. *JACC Cardiovasc Imaging.* 9:1367–1376, 2016.

Lincoln AE, Vogel RA, Allen TW, et al. Risk and Causes of Death Among Former National Football League Players (1986–2012). *Med Sci Sports Exerc.* 50:486–493, 2018.

Lynall RC, Kerr ZY, Parr MS, et al. Division I College Football Concussion Rates Are Higher at Higher Altitudes. *J Orthop Sports Phys Ther.* 46:96–103, 2016.

Lynall RC, Pietrosimone B, Kerr ZY, et al. Osteoarthritis Prevalence in Retired National Football League Players With a History of Concussion and Lower Extremity Injury. *J Athl Train.* 52:518–525, 2017.

Maher JT, Levine PH, Cymerman A. Human Coagulation Abnormalities During Acute Exposure to Hypobaric Hypoxia. *J Appl Physiol.* 41:702–707, 1976.

Marchi N, Bazarian JJ, Puvenna V, et al. Consequences of Repeated Blood-Brain Barrier Disruption in Football Players. *PLoS One.* 8:e56805, 2013.

Marchi N, Cavaglia M, Fazio V, et al. Peripheral Markers of Blood-Brain Barrier Damage. *Clin Chim Acta.* 342:1–12, 2004.

Matveev, LP. *Sport Training Periodization* [in Russian]. Teor Pratk Fiz Kult: Moscow, 1958.

Mayhew JL, Levy B, McCormick T, et al. Strength Norms for NCAA Division II College Football Players. *NSCA J.* 9:67–69, 1987.

Mayhew JL, Ware JS, Bemben MG, et al. The NFL-225 Test as a Measure of Bench Press Strength in College Football Players. *J Strength Cond Res.* 13:130–134, 1999.

McCrea M, Broglio SP, McAllister TW, et al. Association of Blood Biomarkers With Acute Sport-Related Concussion in Collegiate Athletes: Findings From the NCAA and Department of Defense CARE Consortium. *JAMA Netw Open.* 3(1):e1919771, 2020.

McCrea M, Guskiewicz KM, Marshall SW, et al. Acute Effects and Recovery Time Following Concussion in Collegiate Football Players: The NCAA Concussion Study. *JAMA.* 290:2556–2563, 2003.

McCullough EA, Kenney WL. Thermal Insulation and Evaporative Resistance of Football Uniforms. *Med Sci Sports Exerc.* 35:832–837, 2003.

McDermott BP, Casa DJ, Ganio MS, et al. Acute Whole-Body Cooling for Exercise-Induced Hyperthermia: A Systematic Review. *J Athl Train.* 44:84–93, 2009.

McGee KJ, Burkett LN. The National Football League Combine: A Reliable Predictor of Draft Status? *J Strength Cond Res.* 17:6–11, 2003.

McKee AC, Gavett BE, Stern RA, et al. TDP-43 Proteinopathy and Motor Neuron Disease in Chronic Traumatic Encephalopathy. *J Neuropathol Exp Neurol.* 69:918–929, 2010.

McKee AC, Stern RA, Nowinski CJ, et al. The Spectrum of Disease in Chronic Traumatic Encephalopathy. *Brain.* 136:43–64, 2013.

Melvin MN, Smith-Ryan AE, Wingfield HL, et al. Muscle Characteristics and Body Composition of NCAA Division I Football Players. *J Strength Cond Res.* 28:3320–3329, 2014.

Mez J, Daneshvar DH, Kiernan PT, et al. Clinicopathological Evaluation of Chronic Traumatic Encephalopathy in Players of American Football. *JAMA.* 318:360–370, 2017.

Miller KC, Long BC, Edwards J. Necessity of Removing American Football Uniforms From Humans With Hyperthermia Before Cold-Water Immersion. *J Athl Train.* 50:1240–1246, 2015.

Miller MA, Croft LB, Belanger AR, et al. Prevalence of Metabolic Syndrome in Retired National Football League Players. *Am J Cardiol.* 101:1281–1284, 2008.

Miller SL, Tipton KD, Chinkes DL, et al. Independent and Combined Effects of Amino Acids and Glucose After Resistance Exercise. *Med Sci Sports Exerc.* 35:449–455, 2003.

Miller TA, White ED, Kinley KA, et al. The Effects of Training History, Player Position, and Body Composition on Exercise Performance in Collegiate Football Players. *J Strength Cond Res.* 16:44–49, 2002.

Minard D. Prevention of Heat Casualties in Marine Corps Recruits. *Mil Med.* 126:261–272, 1961.

Mitchell G. DLA Piper US LLP. *Report to the Commissioner of Baseball of an Independent Investigation into the Illegal Use of Steroids and Other Performance Enhancing Substances by Players in Major League Baseball,* December 13, 2007.

Montgomery JC, MacDonald JA. Effects of Temperature on Nervous System: Implications for Behavioral Performance. *Am J Physiol: Reg Integ Comp Phys.* 259:R191–R196, 1990.

Moore DR, Areta J, Coffey VG, et al. Daytime Pattern of Post-Exercise Protein Intake Affects Whole-Body Protein Turnover in Resistance-Trained Males. *Nutr Metab.* 9(1):91, 2012.

Moore DR, Robinson MJ, Fry JL, et al. Ingested Protein Dose Response of Muscle and Albumin Protein Synthesis After Resistance Exercise in Young Men. *Am J Clin Nutr.* 89:161–168, 2009.

Mujika I, Halson S, Burke LM, et al. An Integrated, Multifactorial Approach to Periodization for Optimal Performance in Individual and Team Sports. *Int J Sports Physiol Perform.* 13:538–561, 2018.

Myer GD, Smith D, Barber Foss KD, et al. Rates of Concussion Are Lower in National Football League Games Played at Higher Altitudes. *J Orthop Sports Phys Ther.* 44:164–172, 2014.

Nassis GP. Effect of Altitude on Football Performance: Analysis of the 2010 FIFA World Cup Data. *J Strength Cond Res.* 27:703–707, 2013.

Nguyen TV, Jayaraman A, Quaglino A, et al. Androgens Selectively Protect Against Apoptosis in Hippocampal Neurones. *J Neuroendocrinol.* 22:1013–1022, 2010.

Nicholas SJ, Nicholas JA, Nicholas C, et al. The Health Status of Retired American Football Players: Super Bowl III Revisited. *Am J Sports Med.* 35:1674–1679, 2007.

Nissen SL, Abumrad NN. Nutritional Role of the Leucine Metabolite Beta-Hydroxy Beta-Methylbutyrate (HMB). *J Nutr Biochem.* 8:300–311, 1997.

Noakes TD. Fluid Replacement During Exercise. *Exerc Sport Sci Rev.* 21:297–330, 1993.

Noel MB, VanHeest JL, Zaneteas P, et al. Body Composition in Division I Football Players. *J Strength Cond Res.* 17:228–237, 2003.

O'Brien C, Castellani JW, Sawka MN. Thermal Face Protection Delays Finger Cooling and Improves Thermal Comfort During Cold Air Exposure. *Eur J Appl Physiol Occup Physiol.* 111:3097–3105, 2011.

O'Carroll RE, MacLeod D. Moderate Altitude Has No Effect on Choice Reaction Time in International Rugby Players. *Br J Sports Med.* 31:151–152, 1997.

O'Connor KL, Baker MM, Dalton SL, et al. Epidemiology of Sport-Related Concussions in High School Athletes: National Athletic Treatment, Injury and Outcomes Network (NATION), 2011–2012 Through 2013–2014. *J Athl Train.* 52:175–185, 2017.

Oliver JM, Anzalone AJ, Stone JD, et al. Fluctuations in Blood Biomarkers of Head Trauma in NCAA Football Athletes Over the Course of a Season. *J Neurosurg.* 29:1–8, 2019.

Oliver JM, Jones MT, Anzalone AJ, et al. A Season of American Football Is Not Associated With Changes in Plasma Tau. *J Neurotrauma.* 34:3295–3300, 2017.

Opplert J, Babault N. Acute Effects of Dynamic Stretching on Muscle Flexibility and Performance: An Analysis of the Current Literature. *Sports Med.* 48:299–325, 2018.

Oris C, Pereira B, Durif J, et al. The Biomarker S100B and Mild Traumatic Brain Injury: A Meta-Analysis. *Pediatrics.* 141(6):e20180037, 2018.

Owens MF, Roach MA. Decision-Making on the Hot Seat and the Short List: Evidence From College Football Fourth Down Decisions. *J Eco Behav Org.* 148:301–314, 2018.

Packer L. Oxidants, Antioxidant Nutrients and the Athlete. *J Sports Sci.* 15:353–363, 1997.

Palumbo S, Mariotti V, Iofrida C, et al. Genes and Aggressive Behavior: Epigenetic Mechanisms Underlying Individual Susceptibility to Aversive Environments. *Front Behav Neurosci.* 12:117, 2018.

Parsons JT, Anderson SA, Casa DJ, et al. Preventing Catastrophic Injury and Death in Collegiate Athletes: Interassociation Recommendations Endorsed by 13 Medical and Sports Medicine Organisations. *J Athl Train.* 54:843–851, 2019.

Pellman EJ, Powell JW, Viano DC, et al. Concussion in Professional Football: Epidemiological Features of Game Injuries and Review of the Literature – Part 3. *Neurosurgery.* 54:81–94, 2004.

Petersson A, Garle M, Holmgren P, et al. Toxicological Findings and Manner of Death in Autopsied Users of Anabolic Androgenic Steroids. *Drug Alcohol Depend.* 81:241–249, 2006.

Phillips SM, Tipton KD, Aarsland A, et al. Mixed Muscle Protein Synthesis and Breakdown After Resistance Exercise in Humans. *Am J Physiol, Endocr Metab.* 273:E99–E107, 1997.

Plisk S, Gambetta V. Tactical Metabolic Training, Part I. *Strength Cond.* 19:44–53, 1997.

Powers SK, Nelson WB, Hudson MB. Exercise-Induced Oxidative Stress in Humans: Cause and Consequences. *Free Radic Biol Med.* 51:942–950, 2011.

Pryor JL, Huggins RA, Casa DJ, et al. A Profile of a National Football League Team. *J Strength Cond Res.* 28:7–13, 2014.

Ransone J, Neighbors K, Lefavi R, et al. The Effect of Beta-Hydroxy Beta-Methylbutyrate on Muscular Strength and Body Composition in Collegiate Football Players. *J Strength Cond Res.* 17:34–39, 2003.

Rawson ES, Dolan E, Saunders B, et al. Creatine Supplementation in Sport, Exercise and Health. In Hoffman JR (ed) *Dietary Supplementation in Sport and Exercise.* Routledge, Taylor and Francis Group, New York, NY, 141–164, 2019.

Rebolledo BJ, Bernard JA, Werner BC, et al. The Association of Vitamin D Status in Lower Extremity Muscle Strains and Core Muscle Injuries at the National Football League Combine. *Arthroscopy.* 34:1280–1285, 2018.

Riley DO, Robbins CA, Cantu RC, et al. Chronic Traumatic Encephalopathy: Contributions From the Boston University Center for the Study of Traumatic Encephalopathy. *Brain Inj.* 29:154–163, 2015.

Rittenberg A, VanHaaren T. *Timeline: Everything That Led to DJ Durkin's Firing at Maryland*, November 1, 2018. www.espn.com/college-football/story/_/id/24351869/maryland-terrapins-football-jordan-mcnair-death-dj-durkin-scandal-line. Accessed April 25, 2020.

Rivlin M, King M, Kruse R, et al. Frostbite in an Adolescent Football Player: A Case Report. *J Athl Train.* 49:97–101, 2014.

Robbins DW, Goodale TL, Kuzmits FE, et al. Changes in the Athletic Profile of Elite College American Football Players. *J Strength Cond Res.* 27:861–874, 2013.

Roberts AL, Pascual-Leone A, Speizer FE, et al. Exposure to American Football and Neuropsychiatric Health in Former National Football League Players: Findings From the Football Players Health Study. *Am J Sports Med.* 47:2871–2880, 2019.

Roberts M, Debeliso M. Olympic Lifting vs. Traditional Lifting Methods for North American High School Football Players. *Turk J Kinesiol.* 4:91–100, 2018.

Rodriguez NR, DiMarco NM, Langley S. Nutrition and Athletic Performance: Position Stand of the American College of Sports Medicine, American Dietetics Association and Dieticians of Canada. *Med Sci Sports Exerc.* 41:709–731, 2009.

Rogatzki MJ, Keuler SA, Harris AE, et al. Response of Protein S100B to Playing American Football, Lifting Weights, and Treadmill Running. *Scand J Med Sci Sports.* 28:2505–2514, 2018.

Rogatzki MJ, Soja SE, McCabe CA, et al. Biomarkers of Brain Injury Following an American Football Game: A Pilot Study. *Int J Immunopathol Pharmacol.* 29:450–457, 2016.

Rome LC. Influence of Temperature on Muscle Recruitment and Muscle Function In Vivo. *Am J Physiol: Reg Integ Comp Phys.* 259:R210–R222, 1990.

Rothaug M, Becker-Pauly C, Rose-John S. The Role of Interleukin-6 Signaling in Nervous Tissue. *Biochim Biophys Acta.* 1863:1218–1227, 2016.

Roy BD, Fowles JR, Hill R, et al. Macronutrient Intake and Whole Body Protein Metabolism Following Resistance Exercise. *Med Sci Sports Exerc.* 32:1412–1418, 2000.

Roy J, Forest G. Greater Circadian Disadvantage During Evening Games for the National Basketball Association (NBA), National Hockey League (NHL) and National Football League (NFL) Teams Travelling Westward. *J Sleep Res.* 27:86–89, 2018.

Sargeant A. Effect of Muscle Temperature on Leg Extension Force and Short-Term Power Output in Humans. *Eur J Appl Physiol.* 56:693–698, 1987.

Saunders B, Dolan E. Beta-Alanine Supplementation in Sport, Exercise and Health. In Hoffman JR (ed) *Dietary Supplementation in Sport and Exercise.* Routledge, Taylor and Francis Group: New York, NY, 117–140, 2019.

Savica R, Parisi JE, Wold LE, et al. High School Football and Risk of Neurodegeneration: A Community-Based Study. *Mayo Clin Proc.* 87:335–340, 2012.

Sawka MA, Young AJ. Physical Exercise in Hot and Cold Climates. In Garrett WE, Kirkendall DT (eds) *Exercise and Sport Science*. Lippincott Williams and Wilkins: Philadelphia, PA, 385–400, 2000.

Sawka MN, Pandolf KB. Effects of Body Water Loss on Physiological Function and Exercise Performance. In Gisolfi CV, Lamb DR (eds) *Fluid Homeostasis During Exercise: Perspectives in Exercise Science and Sports Medicine*. Vol. 3. Benchmark Press: Indianapolis, 1–38, 1990.

Sawyer DT, Ostarello JZ, Suess EA, et al. Relationship Between Football Playing Ability and Selected Performance Measures. *J Strength Cond Res*. 16:611–616, 2002.

Schmidt WD. Strength and Physiological Characteristics of NCAA Division III American Football Players. *J Strength Cond Res*. 13:210–213, 1999.

Schulte S, Podlog LW, Hamson-Utley JJ, et al. A Systematic Review of the Biomarker S100B: Implications for Sport-Related Concussion Management. *J Athl Train*. 49(6):830–850, 2014.

Schwenk TL, Gorenflo DW, Dopp RR, et al. Depression and Pain in Retired Professional Football Players. *Med Sci Sports Exerc*. 39:599–605, 2007.

Scott CW, Klika AB, Lo MM, et al. Tau Protein Induces Bundling of Microtubules In Vitro: Comparison of Different Tau Isoforms and a Tau Protein Fragment. *J Neurosci Res*. 33:19–29, 1992.

Secora CA, Latin RW, Berg KE, et al. Comparison of Physical and Performance Characteristics of NCAA Division I Football Players: 1987 and 2000. *J Strength Cond Res*. 18:286–291, 2004.

Selakovic D, Joksimovic J, Zaletel I, et al. The Opposite Effects of Nandrolone Decanoate and Exercise on Anxiety Levels in Rats May Involve Alterations in Hippocampal Parvalbumin-Positive Interneurons. *PLoS One*. 12(12):e0189595, 2017.

Shankar PR, Fields SK, Collins CL, et al. Epidemiology of High School and Collegiate Football Injuries in the United States, 2005–2006. *Am J Sports Med*. 35:1295–1303, 2007.

Shields CL, Whitney FE, Zomar VD. Exercise Performance of Professional Football Players. *Am J Sports Med*. 12:455–459, 1984.

Short SH, Short WR. Four-Year Study of University Athletes' Dietary Intake. *J Am Diet Assoc*. 82:632, 1983.

Shrey DW, Griesbach GS, Giza CC. The Pathophysiology of Concussions in Youth. *Phys Med Rehabil Clin N Am*. 22:577–602, 2011.

Shurley JP, Todd JS. "The Strength of Nebraska": Boyd Epley, Husker Power, and the Formation of the Strength Coaching Profession. *J Strength Cond Res*. 26:3177–3188, 2012.

Shurley JP, Todd JS, Todd TC. The Science of Strength: Reflections on the National Strength and Conditioning Association and the Emergence of Research-Based Strength and Conditioning. *J Strength Cond Res*. 31:517–530, 2017.

Siedler DG, Chuah MI, Kirkcaldie MT, et al. Diffuse Axonal Injury in Brain Trauma: Insights From Alterations in Neurofilaments. *Front Cell Neurosci*. 8:429, 2014.

Sierer SP, Battaglini CL, Mihalik JP, et al. The National Football League Combine: Performance Differences Between Drafted and Nondrafted Players Entering the 2004 and 2005 Drafts. *J Strength Cond Res*. 22:6–12, 2008.

Siman R, Shahim P, Tegner Y, et al. Serum SNTF Increases in Concussed Professional Ice Hockey Players and Relates to the Severity of Post-Concussion Symptoms. *J Neurotrauma*. 32:1294–1300, 2015.

Simon JE, Docherty CL. Current Health-Related Quality of Life in Former National Collegiate Athletic Association Division I Collision Athletes Compared With Contact and Limited-Contact Athletes. *J Athl Train*. 51:205–212, 2016.

Singh MV, Rawal SB, Tyagi AK. Body Fluid Status on Induction, Reinduction and Prolonged Stay at High Altitude on Human Volunteers. *Int J Biomet*. 34:93–97, 1990.

Sjogaard, G. Water and Electrolyte Fluxes During Exercise and Their Relation to Muscle Fatigue. *Acta Physiol Scand*. 128(supp):129–136, 1986.

Smith DW, Myer GD, Currie DW, et al. Altitude Modulates Concussion Incidence: Implications for Optimizing Brain Compliance to Prevent Brain Injury in Athletes. *Orthop J Sports Med*. 1(6). doi:10.1177/2325967113511588, 2013.

Smith JF, Mansfield ER. Body Composition Prediction in University Football Players. *Med Sci Sports Exerc*. 16:398–405, 1984.

Smith RA, Martin GJ, Szivak TK, et al. The Effects of Resistance Training Prioritization in NCAA Division I Football Summer Training. *J Strength Cond Res*. 28:14–22, 2014.

Smoot MK, Cavanaugh JE, Amendola A, et al. Creatine Kinase Levels During Preseason Camp in National Collegiate Athletic Association Division I Football Athletes. *Clin J Sport Med*. 24:438–440, 2014.

Snow TK, Millard-Stafford M, Rosskopf LB. Body Composition Profile of NFL Football Players. *J Strength Cond Res*. 12:146–149, 1998.

Song SK, Sun SW, Ramsbottom MJ, et al. Dysmyelination Revealed Through MRI as Increased Radial (but Unchanged Axial) Diffusion of Water. *Neuroimage*. 17:1429–1436, 2002.

Song SK, Wikstrom EA, Tennant JN, et al. Osteoarthritis Prevalence in Retired National Football League Players With a History of Ankle Injuries and Surgery. *J Athl Train*. 54:1165–1170, 2019.

Spotrac website. www.spotrac.com/nfl/draft/. Accessed March 24, 2020.

Spriet LL. Caffeine and Performance. *Int J Sports Nutr*. 5:S84–S99, 1995.

Stamm JM, Koerte IK, Muehlmann M, et al. Age at First Exposure to Football Is Associated With Altered Corpus Callosum White Matter Microstructure in Former Professional Football Players. *J Neurotrauma*. 32:1768–1776, 2015.

Stamp J. *Leatherhead to Radio-Head: The Evolution of the Football Helmet*, 2012. www.smithsonianmag.com/arts-culture/leatherhead-to-radio-head-the-evolution-of-the-football-helmet-56585562/. Accessed April 1, 2020.

Stanley J, Peake JM, Buchheit M. Cardiac Parasympathetic Reactivation Following Exercise: Implications for Training Prescription. *Sports Med*. 43:1259–1277, 2013.

Stein RB, Gordon T, Shriver J. Temperature Dependence of Mammalian Muscle Contractions and ATPase Activities. *J Biophys*. 40:97–107, 1982.

Steiner ME, Berkstresser BD, Richardson L, et al. Full-Contact Practice and Injuries in College Football. *Sports Health*. 8:217–223, 2016.

Stodden DF, Galitski HM. Longitudinal Effects of a Collegiate Strength and Conditioning Program in American Football. *J Strength Cond Res*. 24:2300–2308, 2010.

Stone JD, Kreutzer A, Mata JD, et al. Changes in Creatine Kinase and Hormones Over the Course of an American Football Season. *J Strength Cond Res*. 33:2481–2487, 2019.

Stone MH, O'Bryant H, Garhammer J. A Hypothetical Model of Strength Training. *J Sports Med*. 21:342–351, 1981.

Stover EA, Zachwieja J, Stofan J, et al. Consistently High Urine Specific Gravity in Adolescent American Football Players and the Impact of an Acute Drinking Strategy. *Int J Sports Med*. 27:330–335, 2006.

Strain J, Didehbani N, Cullum CM, et al. Depressive Symptoms and White Matter Dysfunction in Retired NFL Players With Concussion History. *Neurology*. 81:25–32, 2013.

Stuempfle KJ, Katch FI, Petrie DF. Body Composition Relates Poorly to Performance Tests in NCAA Division III Football Players. *J Strength Cond Res*. 17:238–244, 2003.

Sun X, Cao ZB, Tanisawa K, et al. Association of Serum 25-Hydroxyvitamin D Concentrations With Glucose Profiles in Male Collegiate Football Athletes. *Int J Sport Nutr Exerc Metab*. 29:420–425, 2019.

Swietach P, Youm JB, Saegusa N, et al. Coupled Ca2+/H+ Transport by Cytoplasmic Buffers Regulates Local Ca2+ and H+ Ion Signaling. *Proc Natl Acad Sci USA*. 110:E2064–E2073, 2013.

Tarazi A, Tator CH, Wennberg R, et al. Motor Function in Former Professional Football Players With History of Multiple Concussions. *J Neurotrauma*. 35:1003–1007, 2018.

Tarnopolsky MA. Caffeine and Endurance Performance. *Sports Med*. 18:109–125, 1994.

Teramoto M, Cross CL, Willick SE. Predictive Value of National Football League Scouting Combine on Future Performance of Running Backs and Wide Receivers. *J Strength Cond Res*. 30:1379–1390, 2016.

Terrell TR, Abramson R, Barth JT, et al. Genetic Polymorphisms Associated With the Risk of Concussion in 1056 College Athletes: A Multicentre Prospective Cohort Study. *Br J Sports Med*. 52:192–198, 2018.

Tipton KD, Ferrando AA, Phillips SM, et al. Postexercise Net Protein Synthesis in Human Muscle From Orally Administered Amino Acids. *Am J Physiol, Endocr Metab*. 276:E628–E634, 1999.

Todd T. Al Roy: Mythbreaker. *Iron Game History*. 2:12–16, 1992.

Toner MM, McArdle WD. Physiological Adjustments of Man to the Cold. In Pandolf KB, Sawka MN, Gonzalez RR (eds) *Human Performance Physiology and Environmental Medicine at Terrestrial Extremes*. Benchmark Press: Indianapolis, 361–399, 1988.

Toner MM, Sawka MN, Foley ME, et al. Effects of Body Mass and Morphology on Thermal Responses in Water. *J Appl Physiol*. 60:521–525, 1986.

Townsend JR. β-Hydroxy-β-Methylbutyrate. In Hoffman JR (ed) *Dietary Supplementation in Sport and Exercise*. Routledge, Taylor and Francis Group: New York, NY, 89–116, 2019.

Trexler ET, Smith-Ryan AE, Defreese JD, et al. Associations Between BMI Change and Cardiometabolic Risk in Retired Football Players. *Med Sci Sports Exerc.* 50:684–690, 2018.

Trexler ET, Smith-Ryan AE, Mann JB, et al. Longitudinal Body Composition Changes in NCAA Division I College Football Players. *J Strength Cond Res.* 31:1–8, 2017.

Trombley PQ, Horning MS, Blakemore LJ. Interactions Between Carnosine and Zinc and Copper: Implications for Neuromodulation and Neuroprotection. *Biochemistry (Mosc).* 65:807–816, 2000.

Tucker AM, Vogel RA, Lincoln AE, et al. Prevalence of Cardiovascular Disease Risk Factors Among National Football League Players. *JAMA.* 301:2111–2119, 2009.

Uberoi A, Sadik J, Lipinski MJ, et al. Association Between Cardiac Dimensions and Athlete Lineup Position: Analysis Using Echocardiography in NCAA Football Team Players. *Phys Sportsmed.* 41:58–66, 2013.

Varanoske AN, Stout JR, Hoffman JR. Effects of β-Alanine Supplementation and Intramuscular Carnosine Content on Exercise Performance and Health. In Bagchi D, Nair S, Sen CK (eds) *Nutrition and Enhanced Sports Performance: Muscle Building, Endurance, and Strength.* 2nd Edition. Elsevier: Amsterdam, 325–345, 2018.

Veicteinas A, Ferretti G, Rennie DW. Superficial Shell Insulation in Resting and Exercising Men in Cold Water. *J Appl Physiol.* 52:1557–1564, 1982.

Vogel JA, Harris CW. Cardiopulmonary Responses of Resting Man During Early Exposure to High Altitude. *J Appl Physiol.* 22:1124–1128, 1967.

Ward MP, Milledge JS, West JB. *High Altitude Medicine and Physiology.* Chapman and Hall Medical: Amsterdam, 1995.

Warren GL, Park ND, Maresca RD, et al. Effect of Caffeine In-Gestion on Muscular Strength and Endurance: A Meta-Analysis. *Med Sci Sport Exerc.* 42:1375–1387, 2010.

Webster S, Rutt R, Weltman A. Physiological Effects of a Weight Loss Regimen Practiced by College Wrestlers. *Med Sci Sports Exerc.* 22:229–234, 1990.

Weiner RB, Wang F, Isaacs SK, et al. Blood Pressure and Left Ventricular Hypertrophy During American-style Football Participation. *Circulation.* 128:524–531, 2013.

Weissberg I, Veksler R, Kamintsky L, et al. Imaging Blood-Brain Barrier Dysfunction in Football Players. *JAMA Neurol.* 71:1453–1445, 2014.

Wellman AD, Coad SC, Flynn PJ, et al. Comparison of Preseason and In-Season Practice and Game Loads in National Collegiate Athletic Association Division I Football Players. *J Strength Cond Res.* 33:1020–1027, 2019.

Wellman AD, Coad SC, Goulet GC, et al. Quantification of Competitive Game Demands of NCAA Division I College Football Players Using Global Positioning Systems. *J Strength Cond Res.* 30:11–19, 2016.

Wells AJ. Caffeine. In Hoffman JR (ed) *Dietary Supplementation in Sport and Exercise.* Routledge, Taylor and Francis Group: New York, NY, 206–232, 2019.

Wenger CB. Human Heat Acclimatization. In Pandolf KB, Sawka MN, Gonzalez RR (eds) *Human Performance Physiology and Environmental Medicine at Terrestrial Extremes.* Benchmark Press: Indianapolis, 153–198, 1988.

Werner EN, Guadagni AJ, Pivarnik JM. Assessment of Nutrition Knowledge in Division I College Athletes. *J Am Coll Health.* 2:1–8, 2020.

Westermann RW, Kerr ZY, Wehr P, et al. Increasing Lower Extremity Injury Rates Across the 2009–2010 to 2014–2015 Seasons of National Collegiate Athletic Association Football: An Unintended Consequence of the "Targeting" Rule Used to Prevent Concussions? *Am J Sports Med.* 44:3230–3236, 2016.

Wilder N, Deivert RG, Hagerman F, et al. The Effects of Low-Dose Creatine Supplementation Versus Creatine Loading in Collegiate Football Players. *J Athl Train.* 36:124–129, 2001.

Wilder N, Gilders R, Hagerman F, et al. The Effects of a 10-Week, Periodized, Off-Season Resistance-Training Program and Creatine Supplementation Among Collegiate Football Players. *J Strength Cond Res.* 16:343–352, 2002.

Wilkinson DJ, Hossain T, Hill DS, et al. Effects of Leucine and Its Metabolite Beta-Hydroxy-Beta-Methylbutyrate on Human Skeletal Muscle Protein Metabolism. *J Physiol.* 591:2911–2923, 2013.

Williams TD, Tolusso DV, Fedewa MV, et al. Comparison of Periodized and Non-Periodized Resistance Training on Maximal Strength: A Meta-Analysis. *Sports Med.* 47:2083–2100, 2017.

Wilmore JH, Haskell WL. Body Composition and Endurance Capacity of Professional Football Players. *J Appl Phys.* 33:564–567, 1972.

Woolf K, Bidwell WK, Carlson AG. Effect of Caffeine as an Ergogenic Aid During Anaerobic Exercise Performance in Caffeine Naïve Collegiate Football Players. *J Strength Cond Res.* 23:1363–1369, 2009.

Wright JA. *Fourth Down Decisions in NFL Football: A Statistical Analysis.* Master's Thesis, California State University, Northridge, 2007.

Wright JE, Vogel JA, Sampson JB, et al. Effects of Travel Across Time Zones (Jet-Lag) on Exercise Capacity and Performance. *Aviat Space Environ Med.* 54:132–137, 1983.

Wroble RR, Moxley DR. The Effect of Winter Sports Participation on High School Football Players: Strength, Power, Agility, and Body Composition. *J Strength Cond Res.* 15:132–135, 2001.

Yaglou CP, Minard D. Control of Heat Casualties at Military Training Centers. *Arch Indust Health.* 16:302–305, 1957.

Yeargin SW, Casa DJ, Armstrong LE, et al. Heat Acclimatization and Hydration Status of American Football Players During Initial Summer Workouts. *J Strength Cond Res.* 20:463–470, 2006.

Yeargin SW, Casa DJ, Judelson DA, et al. Thermoregulatory Responses and Hydration Practices in Heat-Acclimatized Adolescents During Preseason High School Football. *J Athl Train.* 45:136–146, 2010.

Yeargin SW, Dompier TP, Casa DJ, et al. Epidemiology of Exertional Heat Illnesses in National Collegiate Athletic Association Athletes During the 2009–2010 Through 2014–2015 Academic Years. *J Athl Train.* 54:55–63, 2019.

INDEX

Page numbers in *italics* and **bold** indicate Figures and Tables, respectively.

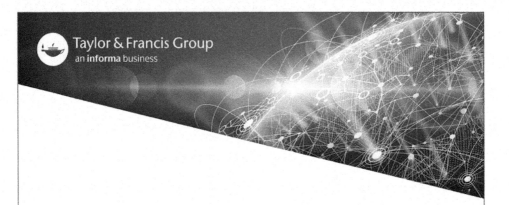
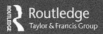
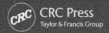

For Product Safety Concerns and Information please contact our EU
representative GPSR@taylorandfrancis.com
Taylor & Francis Verlag GmbH, Kaufingerstraße 24, 80331 München, Germany

www.ingramcontent.com/pod-product-compliance
Ingram Content Group UK Ltd.
Pitfield, Milton Keynes, MK11 3LW, UK
UKHW031041080625
459435UK00013B/568